The Student's Companion
TO Physiotherapy

For Elsevier
Commissioning Editor: Rita Demetriou-Swanwick
Development Editor: Veronika Watkins
Project Manager: Mahalakshmi Nithyanand
Designer/Design Direction: Stewart Larking
Illustration Manager: Gillian Richards
Illustrator: David Banks

THE **Student's Companion** TO **Physiotherapy**

A SURVIVAL GUIDE

edited by

Nick T. Southorn BSc (Hons), MCSP, SRP
Chartered Physiotherapist, Derbyshire, UK

Illustrations by David Banks

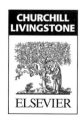

Edinburgh · London · New York · Oxford · Philadelphia · St Louis · Sydney · Toronto 2010

CHURCHILL LIVINGSTONE

ISBN 978-0-7020-3380-3

British Library Cataloguing in Publication Data
A catalogue record for this book is available from the British Library

Library of Congress Cataloging in Publication Data
A catalog record for this book is available from the Library of Congress

Notices
Knowledge and best practice in this field are constantly changing. As new research and experience broaden our understanding, changes in research methods, professional practices, or medical treatment may become necessary.

Practitioners and researchers must always rely on their own experience and knowledge in evaluating and using any information, methods, compounds, or experiments described herein. In using such information or methods they should be mindful of their own safety and the safety of others, including parties for whom they have a professional responsibility.

With respect to any drug or pharmaceutical products identified, readers are advised to check the most current information provided (i) on procedures featured or (ii) by the manufacturer of each product to be administered, to verify the recommended dose or formula, the method and duration of administration, and contraindications. It is the responsibility of practitioners, relying on their own experience and knowledge of their patients, to make diagnoses, to determine dosages and the best treatment for each individual patient, and to take all appropriate safety precautions.

To the fullest extent of the law, neither the Publisher nor the authors, contributors, or editors, assume any liability for any injury and/or damage to persons or property as a matter of products liability, negligence or otherwise, or from any use or operation of any methods, products, instructions, or ideas contained in the material herein.

ELSEVIER your source for books, journals and multimedia in the health sciences

www.elsevierhealth.com

Printed in China

Working together to grow libraries in developing countries

www.elsevier.com | www.bookaid.org | www.sabre.org

ELSEVIER BOOK AID International Sabre Foundation

The Publisher's policy is to use **paper manufactured from sustainable forests**

Contributors   xi
Acknowledgements   xii
Editor's introduction   xiii
An introduction by Professor the Baroness Finlay of Llandaff, MD, FRCP   xiv

Section 1 Settling in

Chapter 1 In the beginning   3

Nick Southorn and Jamie Mackler

Day one   4
What is Physiotherapy?   5
  Definitions vary around the world   5
A brief history of Physiotherapy   5
Physiotherapists at work   7
International organizations   9
Swatting up   9
Books to buy   9
Equipment   10
  Stethoscope   10
  Measuring equipment   11
  Clothing   11
Freshers' week   11
Study tips   13
Being a member of the representative body of Physiotherapy   14
  What is the Chartered Society of Physiotherapy (CSP)?   14
  How to become a student member   14
  Fees (correct as of September 2008)   15
  CSP students' officer   16
  Student representatives   17
  Interactive CSP (iCSP)   17
  Other ways to get involved   18
  CSP networks   18
  Clinical placements   19
  Insurance   19
  Elective placements overseas   19
  Additional funding   19
  References for additional funding   21
  References   21

Chapter 2 Things I wish they'd told me before I started   23

Stuart Porter

What am I letting myself in for?   24
Not sure I deserve to be here   24

Contents

What is different about studying at degree level? 25
The language of the university 25
How to conduct yourself 26
What your lecturers expect from you 27
How do I get through the first year? 30
What you should expect from your lecturers 30
How to get through your exams 31
    Why do students fail? 32
Finally 34

Section 2 Studying physiotherapy

Chapter 3 Anatomy and physiology 37

Nick Southorn

Introduction – anatomy 38
    Visualizing anatomy 38
    Mnemonics and chants 39
    Other methods 40
Introduction – physiology 41
    Learning physiology 41
    "Tool box" 43
In the clinic 43
Conclusion 44
    References 44

Chapter 4 Musculoskeletal physiotherapy 45

Nick Southorn

So *what is* musculoskeletal therapy? 47
Initial subjective assessment 47
Initial objective assessment 50
Clinical semaphore 52
Treatments 52
    Maitland 53
    Cyriax/orthopedic medicine 54
    McKenzie 54
    Acupuncture 54
Muscle energy techniques (MET) 55
    Myofascial therapy 56
    Pilates 56
    Exercise therapy 57

Massage   58
In the clinic   58
References   59

Chapter 5 **Electrotherapy   61**

Tim Watson

What is it?   62
Why is it important?   64
Useful ways to study   64
Resources and information   65
Reference 68

Chapter 6 **Cardiopulmonary physiotherapy   69**

Mandy Jones

Learning the theory   70
Tips for learning anatomy   71
Tips for learning physiology   72
Tips for learning physiotherapy   72
Preparation for clinical placement   73
Tips for clinical placement   75
Hazards of clinical placement   77
Conclusion   79
References   80
Further reading   80

Chapter 7 **Neurologic physiotherapy   81**

Nick Southorn

What you need to know   82
Basics   83
Conditions   85
Assessment   86
Treatment of the neurologic patient   88
In the clinic   90
References   91

Chapter 8 **Pharmacology   93**

Nick Southorn

How do I get my head around all of this?   94
It's all about class!   95

What do I need to know about these drugs?   97
In the clinic   98
Conclusion   98
References   99

Chapter 9 **Biopsychosocial approach**   **101**

Paul Watson

Why a biopsychosocial perspective?   102
A biopsychosocial model of pain disability   103
So what are the important things to consider?   104
In the clinic   107
Integrating assessment into practice   107
Conclusion   109
References   109

Chapter 10 **Pediatrics**   **111**

Nick Southorn

Be a child, it helps!   112
Childhood diseases   113
How to assess a child patient   114
Subjective assessment   114
Objective assessment   115
Treatments   117
Conclusion   118
References   118

Chapter 11 **Clinical placement**   **119**

Nick Southorn

How to prepare   120
What you need to know before you get there   122
Uniform etiquette   122
What you need to know when you get there   126
The learning agreement   128
Marking criteria   128
The role of the clinical educator   130
The role of the academic tutor   131
Conclusion   131
References   132

Section 3 The final stretch

Chapter 12 Clinical audit and research 135

Herbert Thurston

Clinical audit 136
Research 136
   Types of research 137
   Getting started in research 139
   Real-life researchers 140
   Further reading 142

Chapter 13 The degree continues 143

Nick Southorn and Nick Clode

Professional practice 144
Evidence-based practice 145
Portfolio development 147
   What is a CPD portfolio? 147
   Why do I need to keep a CPD portfolio? 148
   What does a portfolio look like? 148
   What should it contain? 149
   Portfolio keeping – what you need to know 149
   Online versus paper-based portfolio systems 151
   Steps in setting up a CPD portfolio 152
   Finally 154
Reflection 154
   References 155
   Further reading 155

Chapter 14 You think it's all over … 157

Nick Southorn and Nick Clode

Results 158
What to do with your textbooks 159
Opportunities for the graduate 159
Looking for jobs in the UK 160
   Websites 161
   Recruitment agencies 162
Interviews 162
   Interview format 163
   Preparation 164
   Interview tips 168

Contents

Appearance 168
On the day 169
Conclusion 170

Index 171

Mike Campbell, BSc (Hons)
Physical Therapist, Toronto, Canada

Nick Clode, BSc (Hons), MCSP
Chartered Physiotherapist, Manchester, UK

Baroness Ilora Finlay of Llandaff, MD, FRCP, FRCGP
Reader/Lecturer in Medicine, Cardiff University College of Medicine, UK
President of the Chartered Society of Physiotherapy

Mandy Jones, PhD, MSc, MCSP, SRP
Senior Lecturer in Cardiopulmonary Physiotherapy, Brunel University, London, UK

Jamie Mackler, BSc (Hons)
Students' Officer, Chartered Society of Physiotherapy, London, UK

Stuart B. Porter, BSc Hons, GradDipPhys, MCSP, SRP, CertMHS
Lecturer in Physiotherapy, University of Salford, UK

Nick T. Southorn, BSc (Hons), MCSP, SRP
Chartered Physiotherapist, Derbyshire, UK

Herbert Thurston, BSc, MBChB(Hons), MD, FRCP
Emeritus Professor of Medicine, the University of Leicester, UK

Paul J. Watson, MSc, PhD, FCSP
Professor of Pain Management and Rehabilitation, Department of Health Sciences, the University of Leicester, UK

Tim Watson, BSc (Hons), PhD, MCSP
Professor of Physiotherapy, University of Hertfordshire, UK

Acknowledgements

My ever-lasting thanks go to each and every student physiotherapist for whom this book is intended. I know that the future of the profession is bright.

The following deserve unlimited thanks for their support over the years.

FAMILY

Special and extensive thanks to my wife, Kate, who supported me throughout physio school and was amazing while I wrote this book by looking after the dogs, horses and goldfish – oh, and all while being pregnant with our first baby! On that, I feel a special thank you should go to Moses Oliver Southorn, my son, who reminds me every day that we have something to smile about, and that sleep isn't necessarily a permanent fixture in one's daily schedule! My parents and my parent-in-laws deserve considerable credit as clearly university would not have been achievable without their continuing support.

FRIENDS

I am grateful to my close friends Mike C, Rik T, Jo P, Sparky, Ceit B, Nick C, Sam H, Jamie M, Lauz C, Shay D, Becki H, Mike O, Mary F and many many more for making physio school so entertaining.

CONTRIBUTORS TO THE BOOK – WHO HENCEFORTH ENTER THE "FRIENDS" CATEGORY

I am indebted to the contributors to this book who not only submitted excellent work but made a distinct effort to maintain friendly contact throughout, which made me feel much better about typing away at times in the morning that I assumed were purely theoretical. Special thanks to Stuart and Mandy whose individual help and advice were invaluable. Neil O'Connell deserves special thanks for his artistic skills. Also, to the guys at Elsevier, Rita D-S and Veronika W, for their belief in this project, wonderful help and friendly banter throughout. Thank you to the scores of people who read and re-read sample chapters and gave help and guidance throughout this project.

Thanks again to Stuart Porter who took photos, provided words of support and wisdom and generally kept me on track. Also a huge acknowledgement to the students of Salford University School of Physiotherapy who appeared in Stuart's photos – Julie Ann Peart modelled expertly for the book, as did Paul Quine, Amy Findlay, Rhian Sunderland and Natalie Earnshaw.

Well, firstly I'd like to say hello and congratulations; you have either been accepted onto a physiotherapy (also known as physical therapy) course or are close to it, so well done! This book is especially for you and I hope that you keep it close by your side throughout the course to graduation day. For the purposes of continuity, I will use the terms "physiotherapy" and "physiotherapist" throughout the text as synonyms for "physical therapy" and "physical therapist" while recognizing and respecting both professional titles.

A lecturer from Nottingham University once said that "one thing that everyone knows about the physiotherapy course is that it is impossible to get on to." This is very true but everything else they know is rarely the full story. Everyone, including health professionals, has their own ideas that have developed from personal experience or hearsay: we either manipulate backs, run onto a football pitch with a "magic sponge" or give out walking frames! The fact is that physiotherapy is a very misunderstood profession and has a much bigger role to play in health than many people believe. It is also possible to get on to the course! I find that one of the most enjoyable aspects of being a physio student is surprising the general public and fellow health professionals with our scope and expertise. This is something that all physio students and all qualified clinicians do naturally and with such aplomb. There will always be orthopedic surgeons who see a respiratory physiotherapist with a stethoscope and conclude that we are listening to joints now! The student has to deal with so many other things too, such as doing well in exams, revision, reading, note taking, impressing clinical educators, etc., and that is why this book exists.

I hope to help you through the process of being a physio student by giving you hints and tips about how to get the most out of being a student. The book will also help you prepare for a variety of key points of the course such as clinical placements, research, continuing professional development (CPD) portfolio development, reflection, etc.

So, this book is for students, written by students (and experts in some cases). It is not prescriptive or a replacement for common sense. Sit back, have a cup of tea and a Kit-Kat and enjoy the course – that, after all, is what university is about.

Nick Southorn, 2009

AN INTRODUCTION BY PROFESSOR THE BARONESS FINLAY OF LLANDAFF, MD, FRCP

Physiotherapy is one of the core healthcare professions. Those entering physiotherapy are high-achieving young people with good academic records and they have a great deal to contribute intellectually through the discipline. The role of the physiotherapist has changed greatly in recent years, taking on more and more of an autonomous practitioner role and often being a key member of a multiprofessional team. In the changing world of rapid rehabilitation to try to get patients home, the physiotherapist's role, in conjunction with occupational therapy, is key. It is the physiotherapist who is able to mobilize the patients, teach patients safe and effective ways of moving and undertaking key tasks, is able to help patients rehabilitate to adapt to their disease process and its treatment and is also able to prevent situations deteriorating by effective interventions such as chest physiotherapy for very sick patients in intensive care units.

The physiotherapy community is developing its own academic research base and has a long-established tradition of high-quality teaching skills.

The intervention of the physiotherapist through teaching patients appropriate musculoskeletal use and ensuring safe and effective respiratory function enables them to maintain independence and enhances a patient's sense of well-being.

The other important role, of course, that the physiotherapist has trained for is rushing onto the sports field and dealing with sporting injuries. In fact, the public image does not recognize the great knowledge and skills involved in a physiotherapist's assessment at the time of an acute injury and the management plan that has to be evolved to allow people to resume normal function after any injury, not only those on the sports field. After road traffic accidents and after major surgery, the physiotherapist becomes essential in restoring patients to active functioning.

Linked to these physical roles is the psychologic well-being that occurs when patients feel more confident and that they have someone who is taking time with them to help address the very real problems that they face. In the future, physiotherapists should have more of a central role in the multiprofessional team and will be vital to allowing hospitals to achieve their throughput targets since they are able to reinforce the well, and also to ensure adaptation to disease and injury.

Section 1
Settling in

You've done the hard bit now… you're in! Now it's time to start enjoying your time as a physio student. No matter where you are in the world, you are joining an exclusive club of special people whose goal in life is to help people (in some cases animals) get better. You are becoming a caring professional and you should be proud. So go out, make friends and have fun!

Chapter 1 **In the beginning** 3

Chapter 2 **Things I wish they'd told me before I started** 23

Section 1

1

In the beginning
Nick Southorn and
Jamie Mackler

- Day one   4
- What is Physiotherapy?   5
- A brief history of Physiotherapy   5
- Physiotherapists at work   7
- International organizations   9
- Swatting up   9
- Books to buy   9
- Equipment   10
- Freshers' week   11
- Study tips   13
- Being a member of the representative
  body of Physiotherapy   14

Settling in

1

Day one

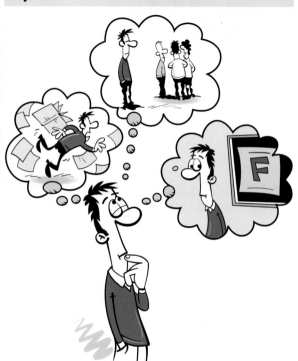

Fig. 1.1 Are you thinking what they are all thinking? Yes, you are!

Nervous? I'm not surprised! Even if you have a degree, starting physio school is nerve racking. "What if I am not clever enough?", "What if I trip in front of everyone in the first lecture?", "Will people like me?" Rest assured that these questions are running through your future friends' minds too so try to relax and be sure to be the first in the lecture theater so if you do trip, nobody will see! The first two chapters of this book will help you feel more at ease.

This chapter aims to give you adequate preparation for starting your degree. There is nothing more embarrassing than when you meet your housemates for the first time and they ask "So, what *is* physiotherapy?" and you have no idea whatsoever – it happens! Some things that *every* student should know is: a brief history of the profession; role of physiotherapists; the name and function of the professional body; and why studying physiotherapy is the best thing in the world (feel free to ad lib for this one!).

What is Physiotherapy?

Physiotherapy practice differs around the globe. In some countries, physiotherapists are clinical doctors; in some countries they offer respiratory therapy; in some countries physiotherapists have little clinical autonomy. However, the physiotherapy profession in general is moving in one direction and with the throughput of ever more determined practitioners, it is hoped that it will continue to prove its effectiveness and necessity in today's modern healthcare environment.

Definitions vary around the world

The American Physical Therapy Association (APTA) defines the physiotherapist as "healthcare professionals who diagnose and treat individuals of all ages, from newborns to the very oldest, who have medical problems or other health-related conditions that limit their abilities to move and perform functional activities in their daily lives" (APTA 2009).

The Canadian Physiotherapy Association (CPA) states that "Physiotherapists manage and prevent many physical problems caused by illness, disease, sport and work related injury, aging, and long periods of inactivity" (CPA 2009).

The Chartered Society of Physiotherapy (CSP), the representative body in the UK, defines physiotherapy as "Physical approaches to promote, maintain and restore physical, psychological and social well-being." They go on to describe physiotherapy as "science-based and committed to extending, applying, evaluating and reviewing the evidence" (CSP 2009).

The New Zealand Society of Physiotherapy (NZSP) states that "Physio-therapists help people move and participate in life and in their communities, especially when movement and function are threatened by ageing, injury, disability or disease" (NZSP 2009).

Basically, physiotherapists are health professionals who assess, diagnose and treat patients using physical and electrotherapeutic modalities including massage, manipulation, acupuncture, percussions, ultrasound, etc. They encourage increased mobility and improved physical fitness by prescription of therapeutic exercises and they practice autonomously (i.e. using their clinical judgment and reasoning and nobody else's). They fill primary care roles or work as part of a health team in a hospital and treat a range of conditions in all types of patients. They also are active researchers and scientists.

Defining physiotherapy with an explanation of the work they do is hard – try to come up with a concise explanation that ticks all the boxes.

A brief history of Physiotherapy

To correctly understand the role of the physiotherapist, one must first look back to where it all began. Only then can it be appreciated how much progress has been made and perhaps gain a little faith that you are joining a dynamic and forward-thinking profession. Physiotherapy as a profession may only be around 110 years old but the techniques we use have been about for literally thousands of years.

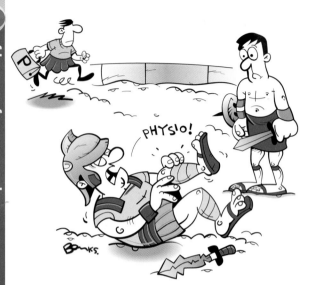

Fig. 1.2 The work of the physiotherapist has been around for thousands of years.

Simple techniques such as massage and even more skillful techniques such as acupuncture are seen as some of the earliest forms of treatment: acupuncture was used over 3000 years ago in China! The so-called "father of medicine," Hippocrates, actually carried out techniques that gave rise to some of the methods we use today. Traction, heat/cryotherapy and manipulation were all practiced by Hippocrates in a crude way over 2000 years ago. The theory was dubious but who cares? It did the job! Of course, in modern-day medicine we have to totally justify *everything* we do by scientific rationale and be *au fait* with the research: this is called "evidence-based practice". Manual techniques over the years were only carried out by physicians but mostly fell away from common usage as medicinal intervention became popular and was more convenient for such a long time. It really began getting busy for "physiotherapists" during the time of the Crimean War (mid 1800s) as rehabilitation specialists for soldiers. A need was established and solidified during the Boer Wars for the same purpose.

Things started looking up for physiotherapy as a profession in 1894 when the "Society of Trained Masseuses" was formed in Great Britain as a professional body to ensure that practitioners were regulated and to avoid the profession falling into disrepute. This was about the time when the professions such as chiropractic and osteopathy were also created. The profession gained more and more momentum around the world with the inception of the Australian Physiotherapy Association in 1906, the provision of physiotherapy training at the University of Otago in New Zealand in 1913 and at Reed College in the United States in 1914. A close working relationship with conventional medicine made sure that physiotherapy was indeed a useful medical profession and thus the British representative body gained a Royal Charter in 1920 and the Physical Therapy Association was formed in 1921 (now known as the American Physical Therapy Association). The current name of the British professional body, the Chartered Society of Physiotherapy (CSP), was adopted in 1944 and the New Zealand Society of Physiotherapists was formed in 1950.

In 1951, countries with developed physiotherapy professions formed the World Confederation of Physical Therapy (WCPT) to enhance world continuity within the profession. More and more training colleges were established and physiotherapy quickly became an integral part of everyday healthcare provision. All around the world, physiotherapy is expanding dramatically; for example, in the early 1980s there were only 10 accredited physiotherapy courses available in India – now there are over 100! Most physiotherapy programs are offered by some of the greatest universities around the world such as Trinity College Dublin, Ireland, the College of Physicians and Surgeons, Columbia University, USA, McGill University, Canada, University of Melbourne, Australia and King's College, London. Physiotherapy is now considered a clinically autonomous profession which assesses, diagnoses and treats a broad range of conditions.

On the whole, then, physiotherapy is a relatively young profession that has forged links and professional relationships with medical treatments, while establishing its own niche as an essential part of everyday "conventional" healthcare provision. We should all be proud of the profession's history and flexibility through the years and look forward to more exciting advances in our working lives and beyond.

Physiotherapists at work

In any hospital you are likely to run into a physiotherapist. They are as settled in primary, secondary and acute care as any physician, surgeon or nurse. The role of the physiotherapist is really quite diverse: you will have the opportunity to work in an emergency department, critical care providing respiratory support, orthopedics/musculoskeletal departments, cardiac rehabilitation, neurologic rehabilitation, amputee care, survivors of torture, women's health, pediatrics, elderly care and so on. In addition to all of this, opportunities are abundant for private clinicians in their own practice: the physiotherapist is seen as the gold standard of sports medical care, and physiotherapists may be employed as personal therapists for someone who requires intensive rehabilitation/physiotherapeutic support.

A surgeon once said of orthopedic physiotherapists that if surgeons make things possible, the physiotherapist makes things happen. This is entirely true in orthopedics – you can't have an ACL reconstruction without the rehab; you can't have a hip replacement without the rehab. Most, if not all, orthopedic surgeries depend upon the skill of the surgeon *and* the physiotherapist. Postsurgical physiotherapy isn't restricted to orthopedics, though – thoracic and abdominal surgery patients need intensive chest physiotherapy, mobility management, scar management and so on.

Increasingly popular nowadays is pain management and vocational rehabilitation for all sorts of chronic conditions. Physiotherapists are adding to their treatment toolkit by becoming increasingly competent at cognitive behavioral therapies (or talking therapy). The idea is to combine standard physiotherapeutic treatments with altering the patient's perception of pain and coping strategies. Physiotherapy has recently been identified as a key factor in return-to-work strategies for people who have had prolonged absence due to illness.

Neurology is another area where physiotherapists are key to rehabilitation, with stroke patients especially. Those who have suffered any sort of neurologic incident, congenital or acquired, traumatic or atraumatic, will need physiotherapy intervention.

Rehab isn't the only trick we have; prevention, or "prehab," is employed by every physiotherapist in terms of pain management, biomechanic/postural education, chest clearance, mobilization of contracted joints, etc. There is little more satisfying than preventing a potentially devastating condition from occurring. An interesting concept is that of the "health coach" whereby the physiotherapist is the point of contact regarding general health maintenance. The idea that one only sees a physio in illness is becoming more outdated as patients like to get regular check-ups for fitness, weight control, diet, relaxation, etc., such as you'd expect with a dentist or optician.

One more area that must be mentioned is veterinary physiotherapy. The veterinary world is increasingly welcoming of animal physiotherapists as more techniques are being proven to be efficient by scientific trial. This is a completely postgraduate area of physiotherapy and therefore not within the scope of this book. For further information on animal physiotherapy, visit www.acpat.org.

So you see that the physiotherapist is more than just a magic sponge-wielding sideline dweller on a sports pitch or an alternative to a chiropractor or osteopath; he or she is an integral cog in healthcare of all conditions in all settings. Whatever the setting, it is expected that as a clinician and a biologic scientist, you are also a potential researcher. Even self-audit is a form of research but more and more physiotherapists are taking dedicated research seriously. It is the researchers in the profession who are ground breaking and highly sought after as they are constantly challenging current trends in order to improve physiotherapy service and evidence base.

They did what? Other roles held by physiotherapists

One of the great aspects of this profession is its versatility; as mentioned above, physiotherapists can be employed by anyone and treat anyone. You will find physiotherapists in nonclinical settings such as equipment sales, advisory roles for production companies, research, some semi-clinical work such as risk assessment, claim assessors, mobility assessors, and then the industrial clinician role of the ergonomic/occupational health expert (also known as "human factor engineers"), e.g. those who work for massive companies designing workstations, treating employees and thinking of ways to cut the number of sick days that the boss has to pay for. More often than not, you will find that a physiotherapist happily combines many of the areas mentioned, providing a well-rounded practitioner. NB: Ergonomics is a profession in its own right; it just so happens that many physiotherapists practice ergonomy due to their detailed understanding of the human body and the effect external stresses have upon it.

International organizations

Wherever you study, there will be a nationwide organizational body that you will belong to on qualifying from physio school. It is advisable to visit the website of the organization early on in your degree as it will provide extremely useful information about your profession. Now is the time to get involved with your organization as you are the future of the profession – better to be prepared.

Swatting up

You may wonder if you should try some preschool reading. It is advisable – but boring. If you do decide to carry this out and prepare yourself academically, you should look at your school's syllabus to see what your first topic is; no point reading up on anatomy if you don't start it for another 6 months. Keep it simple too – you should look at learning basic principals and let your lecturers guide you into more depth as appropriate. Throughout this book you will be guided through the core topics and useful hints are given on how to study each area. Whatever you choose to do, make sure you keep your notes as it is pointless if you don't utilize the progress you make.

Books to buy

You are going to have to buy some books. It is advisable to buy the most recent edition of a book for the simple reason that it will be the most up to date in terms of research, practice and economic climate. There is no true "timeless" text because of advances in research and ways of thinking so even standard anatomy books need updating. In addition to this, buying a new book gives you a real sense of ownership as you can add any notes you wish and not have to erase the previous owner's scribbles.

Although every university has its own reading list, you will definitely be requiring good, solid anatomy, physiology and biomechanics books as well as good pocket books. There are plenty to choose from, for a good reason – everyone has different ways of thinking and learning. On this, I suggest that you head off to a library and sit for the day looking at different anatomy, physiology and biomechanics books and thinking about which author suits you best. Putting in this early work will make studying much more tolerable.

Traditionalists will point you towards *Gray's anatomy* (Standing 2008) as this is closest to the gold standard of anatomy textbooks. However, it is heavy going and relentless in its fact delivery which can induce boredom quite quickly: it is, after all, a reference book rather than a "teaching book." There are also anatomy books out there that, although providing a basic overview, may fall below the standard expected of you as a physiotherapist. The choice is extensive, from the informative and dull to the basic and fun, such as anatomy coloring books; if you keep a good lookout you will come across a text that suits the level that *you* need. Remember that sooner or later you will have to bring your anatomic knowledge up to a very high level as our skill as diagnosticians of physical conditions comes from not only our ability to name each joint, muscle, bone and ligament but identifying its normal and

9

pathologic function. Anatomy is hard work – make it as easy as you can by buying yourself the most suitable book for you.

Physiology books are a tough one too. Again, there are the traditional physiology texts such as *Ganong's review of medical physiology* (Barrett et al 2009) but they are tough reading. Physiology is just as important as a keen knowledge will foster excellent differential diagnostic skills. The advice is the same as for anatomy, I'm afraid: put in the hard work now and you will reap the benefits later. I would advise that you consider a text that makes explicit links to clinical medicine as physiology can sometimes be hard to "make real" when you are looking at things on such a microscopic level.

Biomechanics is a topic that horrifies a lot of people but one that physiotherapists must master. Therefore an approachable book that provides a gentle introduction is a must. *Tidy's physiotherapy* (Porter 2008) is recommended as it introduces biomechanics nicely along with many other areas of physiotherapy.

Elsevier do a nice range of pocket books covering topics from pain (Stannard & Booth 2004) to on-call survival guides (Harden 2004). The most popular book you will find poking out of most physiotherapists' jacket pocket is *The physiotherapist's pocket book* (Kenyon & Kenyon 2009). It is a popular choice because of its Dr Who Tardis characteristic of having far more stuff inside it that its apparent size allows.

If you have a large budget you can go crazy buying very specific books, e.g. books on how to measure joints, how to use a stethoscope, etc. These are fine but remember that skills such as these come from practical learning and listening to what practitioners have to say on the matter.

Many books now also have an interactive element whereby you gain access to a related website (Gray's anatomy for students, Netters anatomy, etc.). These are very useful as you can copy and paste the pictures on to your computer for your own notes.

Equipment

You may get an equipment list from your university that contains things such as a goniometer, tape measure, stethoscope, etc. It is temping to run out and get all of this but you should be aware that a lot of universities run a discount day for these products whereby a local retailer comes in to sell stuff at lower prices. It's worth asking as some of this kit can be expensive.

Stethoscope

The cost of these will range from as little as a pint of beer to the cost of a small second-hand car! Essentially, you need to have a serious think about this purchase. The cheapest will not be comfortable in your ears and will not be sensitive enough to pick up the intricate noises you are expected to hear – plus they look like they came from a play set! However, the most expensive ones are well beyond anything you are likely to need in the next 5 years or so. Whatever you go for, look at the ear pieces – are they plastic or rubber? Are they replaceable? Look at the diaphragm and bell – is it a "floating diaphragm"? Is it appropriate for what you will be using it for (i.e. will you be able to use it on pediatric patients?). Look at the tubing – is it likely to crack/kink/degenerate over the next few years? This is an important buy and one that you should take your time over. More information regarding this purchase can be found in Chapter 6 – Cardiopulmonary physiotherapy.

Measuring equipment

You are welcome to buy your own and it is convenient to do so but things like measuring tape and goniometers are usually provided in hospitals and universities. It all comes down to budget and whether you can find time to hunt this equipment down.

Tape measures are infinitely useful tools. You can measure movements such as spinal flexion and cervical rotation, diameter of a swollen limbs or limb length discrepancies. A soft material is a must and one that can be cleaned with an alcohol wipe after each use. Nice retractable ones are available too but, again, less expensive ones may be prone to short lifespans.

Goniometers are used for joint ranges and vary in size according to the joint to be measured. A 6 or 8 inch model will be sufficient for your needs as they are capable of measuring most joints. Small finger goniometers are available and huge 12 inch versions are available too. They come in a whole range of colors, materials and durabilities but to be honest, a simple clear one will suffice; as long as you can see the numbers and the guide lines, you'll be fine.

Don't get thinking about the long list of specialist tools such as a hand dynamometer, pressure algometer or peak flow meter because you just don't need to buy that stuff (unless your university specifies that you do!).

On the whole, you are a student and as such you have access to your university or hospital equipment so don't sweat it too much!

Clothing

Having researched this, it is apparent that every university has different rules and regulations regarding uniform. Please do adhere to these rules – it's not worth the hassle of trying to challenge them. Whatever your university suggests you wear, remember that you are a professional student and therefore need to look smart and presentable at all times. Look at your introduction pack from your university for further information about clinical clothing.

For practical classes, however, make sure you have appropriate shorts and t-shirts. It is unbelievably common for a physio student to turn up to a lower limb assessment practical with jeans on, having forgotten their shorts. Please don't do this as one of two things will happen: you will be sent away or you will be provided with the dreaded university shorts that have years of experience with forgetful students … and usually the stench to prove it. You'd be rightly annoyed if a patient of yours had inappropriate clothing for the assessment so don't do it to your colleagues!

Freshers' week

Freshers' week is a time for celebration, enjoyment, socializing and making friends. While doing this, don't forget to take the time to explore your new home from home. You may have lectures in freshers' week that explain all about the library, computer systems, chaplaincy, students' union, and other generic university-based facts; you may also get some course-specific ones too. These can be tediously dull but remember that the person giving the lecture is there to make your life easier. All you will do is end up asking for help if you don't listen. Also, the person giving the lecture may not be a lecturer but an administrator so forgive them if they don't capture your imagination when talking about computer programming or filing systems in the library.

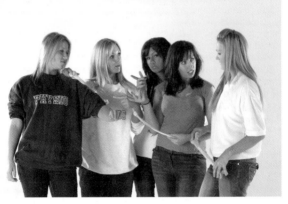

Fig. 1.3 You'll make new friends pretty quickly at physio school and before you know it, you'll find yourself talking "physio" most of the time.

Littering is never acceptable

Freshers' week will also see the street full of people handing out leaflets/flyers, etc. and people promptly ditching them a few hundred yards later. Don't be inconsiderate and litter – it is a disgrace to see the streets of a university town after freshers' week so please set an example and put unwanted flyers in the trash or recycling bin.

One huge part of this week is the opportunity for you to join a society, sports club, etc. These are great ways to make friends outside physiotherapy and may be an opportunity to take up a new hobby. Have a look at your university's students' union for further details; remember that if there is a society or sport that doesn't exist yet, you can create one! Not only does it give you a great hobby and sense of responsibility but it looks great to potential employers on your curriculum vitae/résumé.

Get to know the staff too. You will be assigned a tutor and the first week is an ideal time to have a meeting with them. Your tutor will play a huge part throughout the course and maybe write you a reference at the end so a good working relationship is a must.

Study tips

Reading through this, you will see how each learning technique fits into the topic being studied. A popular style is group work. This is advantageous for so many reasons.

- Team-building skills are developed – you will soon discover how you can contribute to a team by doing this.

- Consolidating friendships – some of your closest friends are made at university and that doesn't just mean the guys you go socializing with. You soon will find a large group you love working with, who are as committed as you are and as productive as you are.

- Breakdown of topics – in medicine, large subjects are studied in great detail. Don't try to take it all on – split it down between you.

- Greater variety of resources and learning styles – you won't all rate the same books or equipment so you will have instant access to your mates' stuff if you become a close and trusting team. Also, some smarty may have found the best way to study a particular topic – try it out, you may like it.

- Shared knowledge – it's easy to miss little bits of information when a lecturer has been talking for 2 hours. Not just the academic stuff but the time frames of work, including deadlines, and the depth you need to study to, etc.

It's not all fun all the time though. Some less appealing points …

- You will rely on your mates to pull their weight; if they don't do what they are supposed to do in time, you risk missing that topic in your notes. Also if they don't study to the required depth of detail, you will have to play catch-up.

- Their learning style may be so different from yours that you may not be able to use their notes – not a huge drama but can be annoying.

- Removed locus of control – you may have problems not controlling exactly what you learn.

- Noncontiguous notes – if you like your notes to match and be color coded, etc. then this will be an issue. You can always convert your notes in your own time.

- Scheduling issues – will your diary match theirs?

These points aside, group work teaches you how to cope with other people's idiosyncrasies and methods. This is an important lesson to learn and will prepare you well for the real world of health provision.

Individual study can be beneficial if you are a very independent person, as long as you are clear as to what is expected of you all the time. It is not advisable to study alone all the time as you are bound to lose focus and get bored or distracted. In these times of Facebook and the thing out of the window that was of no interest before but is fascinating all of a sudden, it is easy to be drawn away from work.

Individual working can promote a sense of discipline and scheduling, qualities that will serve you very well as a clinician. Also, you have complete control over your learning and you can explore each topic to the depth you wish as your interest dictates (this is a double-edged sword, though, as you can't hide from neurology forever!).

Never take on too much. It is understandable to have to work to pay bills, etc, but try to be realistic – a good deal of prioritization is needed. This comes from someone who decided his final year would be a good time to write a book!

Ultimately, how you study should meet your needs – you should never feel pressured into an uncomfortable working situation as you will never get a lot from it. If you are desperate to do some group work, you will find plenty of willing volunteers I'm sure.

Student wisdom

"Always make time for hobbies and interests outside of your studies, enabling you to de-stress and switch off."
Suzanne Temple, Nottingham, UK

"It might sound simple but making an effort to keep notes in order and filed away will save lots of time and energy wasted trying to find and eventually having to rewrite them. It's amazing how easy it is to become an untidy student!"
Anon, South Africa

Being a member of the representative body of Physiotherapy

J. Mackler

This section is aimed at British students regarding the membership of the Chartered Society of Physiotherapy. This chapter is worth reading even if you are not a British student as it will give you an idea about what you can expect from your representative body.

What is the Chartered Society of Physiotherapy (CSP)?

The CSP is the professional, educational and trade union of the nearly 50,000 physiotherapists in the United Kingdom. It champions the role of physiotherapy in modern healthcare, supports members at work and fosters professional learning and progression. In real terms for students, it provides a wealth of information regarding professional practice and support for those who need it. It has a student-led system whereby it acts upon the concerns and comments of the student body regarding professional or educational issues. To facilitate this role, it employs a dedicated students' officer.

How to become a student member

Once you are on a UK physiotherapy degree program, you can apply online for CSP student membership by visiting the website www.csp.org.uk (and follow the links to student membership) or by filling out an application form.

Students are seen as a vital part of the CSP membership and are therefore encouraged to participate at all levels within the society, from local branch meetings up to and including the society's Council which is the sovereign body of the organization. In addition, student members also have their own representative structures. There are elected student representatives at each physiotherapy university (one or two for each year), who deal with the issues of student physiotherapists at a local level, and the Students' Executive Committee (SEC), which carries out national student work.

Fees (correct as of September 2008)

CSP student membership costs only £32 per year. For students enrolled on a program without CSP approval, the tariff is £40 per year. To check if a course is approved, please visit the CSP website www.csp.org.

For less than the cost of a pint of lager per month, these are some of the benefits of CSP student membership.

- Your own continuing professional development (CPD) e-portfolio that provides a quick and enjoyable way to keep an ongoing, complete record of your professional skills and knowledge gained throughout your course. This is invaluable for keeping track of placement and university learning and essential for helping prepare job applications and more on graduation.

- Regular copies of *Physiotherapy Frontline* magazine, and access to current and back-copies of *Physiotherapy* journal online, saving money if both bought independently.

- Students' area and access to a wealth of information on the CSP's website www.csp.org.uk, including access to the member-only area.

- Full access to www.interactiveCSP.org.uk where you can find invaluable advice and tips as well as post messages and start discussions with thousands of other users and a dedicated student network.

- *Rules of professional conduct and the core standards for physiotherapy practice* – available to download from the CSP website.

- Regular students' newsletter.

- Use of the CSP Library and Information Service, which exists to support all CSP members with their research and CPD and to support evidence-based practice.

- The new CSP Library Online Public Access Catalogue (OPAC), now available at http://csplis.csp.org.uk, giving you access to its extensive collection of specialist books, journals, reports, theses and CSP publications, much now available for loan either in person or by post.

- A full-time dedicated Students' Officer to co-ordinate student services and help you during your time as a student.

- The CSP's friendly and knowledgeable enquiry staff are at the end of the phone and will assist you or point you in the right direction on all aspects of physiotherapy: 020 7306 6666.

- CSP student membership card and student badge.

- Visits from your Students' Officer and other CSP staff.

- Local, regional and national student representation, carried out by a well-trained network of CSP student reps and student regional co-ordinators who are there to represent all student members' interests.

- Student representation on the CSP Council, Learning and Development, Professional Practice and Industrial Relations Committees.
- Involvement in a national organization with the knowledge that the CSP is campaigning on behalf of physiotherapists and the profession of physiotherapy at local, regional and national level, safeguarding the future of your profession and ensuring the best employment conditions for all physiotherapists.
- The benefit of student PLI – professional and personal liability indemnity insurance. The CSP's insurers have recommended that all students need individualized cover and should not rely on their placement to provide cover for them.
- Joe Jeans Memorial Fund (financial assistance for elective placements overseas).
- Workshops on clinical topics, usually in your first term, for CSP student members only (new members can join on the day and attend workshop).
- Access to join one of over 40 professional network groups with a diverse range of clinical occupational interests, giving you the opportunity to learn more about a particular area of interest, making your CV stand out when applying for your first post.
- In your first year you can stand for election as a CSP student rep and receive induction training and the opportunity to attend the CSP Student Representatives' Conference free of charge.
- The CSP offers a complete online job search service: www.jobescalator.com

CSP students' officer

The CSP employs a full-time Students' Officer to act as a focus point for all student involvement in the society. The Students' Officer keeps in regular

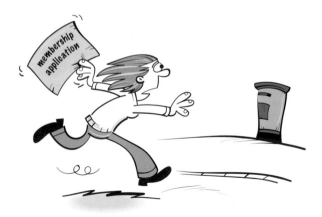

Fig. 1.4 Please get your membership application in as soon as you can.

contact with CSP student representatives at each university, ensuring that effective communication is maintained. The Students' Officer also visits physiotherapy university departments to promote the activities of the society, answer questions and offer advice.

Life as a student is not always as trouble free as some may like to think. CSP student members are free to contact the Students' Officer at any time for help or advice with any aspect of student life. They can also contact their students' union for more localized support. Telephone calls or letters will be treated as confidential on request.

The Students' Officer is based in the Practice and Development function of the CSP. Email: macklerj@csp.org.uk.

Student representatives

Each physiotherapy course has at least one CSP student representative from each year. Representatives act as an important means of communication between student physiotherapists and the CSP, disseminating information at a local level. Representatives also promote the services and information available from the CSP and feed back any problems or concerns facing their colleagues to the Students' Officer.

The annual Student Representatives' Conference is held over a weekend at the end of February. It is funded by the CSP and attended by representatives from each physiotherapy university department in the United Kingdom.

The first morning of the conference is given over to workshops on areas of particular interest. Previous workshops have included pilates, acupuncture and sports physiotherapy. The afternoon provides an opportunity to debate motions on student issues, which have been submitted by student members up and down the country. The results of these motions direct the student work of the CSP for the coming year. The second day includes the election of the new Student Executive Committee (SEC) and regional co-ordinators, and enables representatives to hold the outgoing committee accountable. The Student Representatives' Conference is just one example of how students can have their say in the direction of the society.

The SEC is the national student committee of the society. The committee's function is to represent student physiotherapists within the society and the profession as a whole. Members help to develop policy, organize student campaigns and take forward motions passed at the Student Representatives' Conference. The members are all students elected annually.

The SEC consists of the student Council member as well as the six regional reps and the nationally elected students on the society's two standing committees (Practice and Development and Industrial Relations) and three country reps (Wales, Northern Ireland and Scotland). The President of the SEC is an honorary position of 2 years' duration held by a CSP Council member who has shown an interest in student affairs. The President supports the student members of Council and gives advice from the point of view of an experienced physiotherapist.

Interactive CSP (iCSP)

One easy way to get involved in the CSP is through iCSP. This is an innovative development for members of the society, which uses the internet to enable physiotherapists to connect with each other and share their knowledge. The system is divided into a wide range of networks, each related to a specific aspect of physiotherapy, e.g. a clinical specialty. The idea is that each user joins the networks that are relevant to their needs and interests. Each network includes a range of content sections including news, events, documents, website links and discussions.

As well as being able to access and contribute to other networks, there is a student network which provides a range of resources and information related to being a physiotherapy student. Members can share content and participate in discussions with fellow students.

Other ways to get involved

Throughout the year, many events are organized to ensure the student voice is heard, such as campaigning and lobbying on important issues such as the student loan campaign as well as raising awareness of the issue of graduate employment. The voice of all physiotherapy students is essential in getting messages across.

Fundraising also plays a big role in the life of a physio student. Many students want to give something back to the community and one way of doing this is by getting involved in fundraising activities with the support of the SEC fundraising co-ordinator. It's a great way to meet people, develop professional skills and have fun while bringing much-needed revenue to charities.

CSP networks

There are three recognized CSP networks for all CSP members: LGBT for lesbian, gay, bisexual and transgender members, Black and Minority Ethnic Members Network and AbilityNet for members with disabilities or a health condition which may or may not affect their ability to carry out their job as a physiotherapist. All are open to students. Membership can involve receiving regular newsletters, briefings on legal developments and details of network meetings and other conferences, which may be of interest. The groups also offer peer support for members who are having difficulties, for example coming out at work and becoming disabled or facing racial harassment.

Academic appeals

If situations in a student's personal life are spilling over into their university life, deadlines have been missed or perhaps they are simply not doing very well because of problems outside their academic life, they may be able to appeal against their mark. They must have good reason why their circumstances were not brought forward as extenuating circumstances in the first place.

There are usually two grounds for appeal.

- Extenuating circumstances that have affected your overall ability or ability to meet deadlines.

- There was a material or procedural irregularity in the assessment of your work, i.e. your work was not marked correctly.

Appeals will not be accepted on the grounds that the student considered their efforts to be undermarked or that the student did not understand or was unaware of course or university regulations. That means you cannot challenge marks received because you are unhappy with them. Student members of the CSP have the right to seek advice from their CSP Students' Officer who is there to assist with appeals. They can help interpret course regulations, put together a stronger appeal or even attend formal hearings on behalf of students (if university regulations permit this).

Clinical placements

About one-third of a UK physiotherapy course is clinical education. This is learning that takes place on placements with practicing physiotherapists (known as clinical educators) and their patients, in actual work settings.

These periods of learning are known as clinical placements. The pattern, duration and location of placements will be chosen by the university and some placements may involve a residential spell away from the student's university base.

Insurance

All student members of the CSP are automatically insured with full public and professional liability insurance. The policy covers the student on all clinical placements, including those voluntarily organized in the student's own time. The key condition of the policy is that the student is supervised at all times by a qualified physiotherapist (there are a few interprofessional learning placements where the immediate supervisor may be of another discipline although a physiotherapist will have overall responsibility for the student's placement program). The policy covers the student for £5 million plus all legal costs in any country in the world except the USA, Canada and Australia. Students requiring proof of cover, because their placement supervisor requests it, should also contact the Students' Officer.

Elective placements overseas

Some physiotherapy courses offer students the opportunity to undertake a placement overseas as part of their clinical experience or as an extra opportunity to gain further experience in an unusual setting. The CSP does not co-ordinate these placements. However, information papers outlining the steps you will need to go through in order to arrange a successful elective overseas are available from the Students' Officer.

Scholarships are available to student members of the CSP to help fund the costs of an overseas elective placement through the Joe Jeans Memorial Fund. Funded jointly by the CSP and Forester Health, two application rounds take place each year in the spring and autumn. Application forms and guidance for applicants can be downloaded from the CSP website or the student network of interactive CSP.

Scholarships are not designed to cover the whole cost of a placement and competition can be quite fierce, so you are advised to seek alternative methods of funding your trip as early as possible. For further information contact the CSP Students' Officer.

Additional funding

Access funds and hardship loans are available to help students who are in financial difficulty. They can be used to help with living expenses and course costs including childcare costs, travel, accommodation costs, household

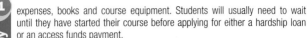
expenses, books and course equipment. Students will usually need to wait until they have started their course before applying for either a hardship loan or an access funds payment.

Colleges decide which students will receive payments and how much each payment will be. Student support or student services staff at universities will be able to advise on how to apply. In some cases students may be able to receive an access fund payment and a hardship loan at the same time.

ACCESS FUNDS

Access funds are available to full-time students, and part-time students studying at least 50% of a full-time course. To qualify, students must meet the same residence conditions as for student loans and be following an undergraduate or postgraduate course. For students who are eligible for a student loan, they must already have applied for their full entitlement before applying to the access funds.

Access funds can be awarded as a short-term loan but are usually paid as a grant. The amounts paid will depend on individual circumstances, how many other applications the university receives and how much is available to give out from access funds each year. Some universities offer bursaries from access funds for mature students and others who might be prevented from completing their course because of financial problems. Bursaries mean students can be awarded a payment for each year of the course and they can apply for help from access funds more than once during the academic year. They will need to give evidence of their financial circumstances for the college to consider their application. Universities decide how to manage their access funds and will deal with any appeals if a student is not satisfied with a decision.

ADDITIONAL GRANTS FROM THE NHS

Some students will be able to apply for additional grants through their NHS bursary. These grants and allowances include the following.

- Dependants' allowances – these are payable to you for people who are wholly or mainly financially dependent on you during your training.
- Single parent addition – you may apply for this allowance if you are a single student who has a dependent child or children.
- There is also a new childcare allowance for NHS students. NHS-funded students are to get help with childcare costs during their studies as part of a new government scheme. The £17 million fund will benefit approximately 6000 students a year, covering up to 85% of childcare costs.
- Clinical placement costs – the travel cost of journeys between your term-time residence and a clinical placement, which is not part of your college, can be reimbursed.

INTEREST-FREE OVERDRAFTS

Most banks will consider existing student account customers for interest-free overdrafts. Most offer about a £400 interest-free overdraft. However, these are not granted automatically so it is worth shopping around to ensure you get the best deal.

References for additional funding

Some organizations offer small amounts of financial assistance to students on specified courses who meet their conditions. You may find these websites of use.

Scholarship Search UK: www.scholarship-search.org.uk

International Education Financial Aid: www.iefa.org

Student Zone: www.studentzone.org.uk

British Council: www.britishcouncil.org/eis/finance.htm

Support 4 Learning: www.support4learning.org.uk

Scorates-ERASMUS: www.europa.eu.int/comm/education/socrates.html

Higher Education Funding Agencies: Scotland: www.student-support-saas.gov.uk;

Wales: www.wales.gov.uk;

Northern Ireland: www.nics.gov.uk;

England: www.dfes.gov.uk/studentsupport

References

American Physical Therapy Association, 2009. About the American Physical Therapy Association. Available at: www.apta.org/AM/Template.cfm?Section=Physical_Therapy&Template=/TaggedPage/TaggedPageDisplay.cfm&TPLID=217&ContentID=34361

Barrett, K.E., Brookes, H., Biotano, S., Barman, S.M. (Eds.), 2009. Ganong's Review of Medical Physiology, twentythird ed. Lange, Connecticut.

Canadian Physiotherapy Association, 2009. Public: about physiotherapy. Available at: www.physiotherapy.ca/public.asp?WCE=C=32IK=S222413

Chartered Society of Physiotherapy, 2009. What is physiotherapy? Available at: www.csp.org.uk/director/public/whatphysiotherapy.cfm.

Harden, B. (Ed.), 2004. Emergency Physiotherapy. Churchill Livingstone, Edinburgh.

Kenyon, J., Kenyon, K., 2009. The Physiotherapist's Pocket Book, second ed. Churchill Livingstone, Edinburgh.

New Zealand Society of Physiotherapy, 2009. Homepage. Available at: www.physiotherapy.org.nz/.

Porter, S. (Ed.), 2008. Tidy's Physiotherapy, fourteenth ed. Chirchill Livingstone, Edinburgh.

Standing, S. (Ed.), 2008. Gray's Anatomy, fortieth ed. Churchill Livingstone, Edinburgh.

Stannard, C., Booth, S., 2004. Pain, second ed. Churchill Livingstone, Edinburgh.

2

Things I wish they'd told me before I started
Stuart Porter

- What am I letting myself in for?   24
- Not sure I deserve to be here   24
- What is different about studying at degree level?   25
- The language of the university   25
- How to conduct yourself   26
- What your lecturers expect from you   27
- How do I get through the first year?   30
- What you should expect from your lecturers   30
- How to get through your exams   31
- Finally   34

Settling in

University brings out all abilities, including incapability.

(Chekhov 1860–1904)

What am I letting myself in for?

You've spent the last few years of your life desperately wanting to be a chartered physiotherapist, you've had careers advisers, parents, partners, physiotherapists and other intelligent and well-informed people telling you what to do, what not to do, and when to do it; that in itself is stressful enough and you've not even started yet! Now you find that you have been offered a place at university and you pass your exams. Then, BANG, you walk into the university on day one and it's suddenly all very real. I hope that this chapter makes your first year a little less stressful.

Not sure I deserve to be here

Also known as "The person sitting next to me looks a lot cleverer than me and she's got A-level biology" syndrome.

I have been a first-year manager for 10 years now and it's a job that I love. It has always been really interesting to watch students comparing themselves with each other. Students do this within minutes of arriving in university on

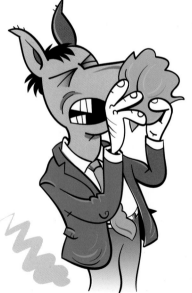

Fig. 2.1 Just relax into university life – try not to worry.

their first day. In psychologic terms this is known as social positioning or social comparison – the phenomenon whereby people compare themselves either positively or negatively with each other. I am not going to go into huge detail about this but what I have found is that people starting a university degree usually view themselves as inferior to their peers; the problem with this is that for many students this persists throughout their entire time at university. I must admit that I tend to do this myself; in my case it is purely a defence mechanism. Here is an exercise for you to complete to show you how common these feelings are in all of us.

We all feel a bit silly sometimes. How many of these did you feel on your first day at university? Tick each that applies to you and be honest.

- Everyone else here is cleverer than me.
- I don't deserve to be here.
- I won't be able to cope with the work.
- What have I let myself in for?
- I can't ask that question, the lecturer will think I'm stupid.
- I'll never be able to remember all this.
- I'll never be as clever as my teachers.

Now see if you can work out who they are based upon in real life.

ANSWER: In September 2000 I enrolled for a PhD. These are the thoughts that went through my mind the first time I met my supervisor. It happens to us all. Stuart Porter.

What is different about studying at degree level?

This is a very important subject so let's make it simple (see Fig. 2.2).

The language of the university

Universities have their own language and culture. You will quickly learn the ground rules for your university and before too long you'll feel like you belong, but in the meantime do not be afraid to ask if you don't understand something. We as academics are apt to forget sometimes that what we think of as a clear rule or term may not be all that clear to you.

During your time at university you may experience some problems that you were not expecting. The key thing to remember is that while you may feel like your world is ending, there is a very good chance that your tutors will have encountered similar problems before and they will know how to advise you or at the very least, they will know who can advise you. The potential problems that you may encounter are too numerous to mention, but examples include financial, psychologic, academic and personal; the key message for all these is that you must let the staff know if you need help. Universities tend to be very understanding if they know in advance of any problems that you have whereas

GCSE level	A level	Degree level
I give you a potato	I give you a potato	I give you a potato
You were expected to give me back the potato. This is parrot fashion recall of facts - you repeat what you have been taught about the potato.	You were expected to go a little deeper and peel the potato. Now there is an element of understanding needed for you to be able to peel the potato.	You were expected to go away and return with a bag of chips, nicely wrapped, with details of how you cooked them and why. To get a first class honours degree, you should go away and study the history of the potato and discuss techniques for cooking them!
		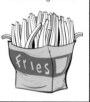

Fig. 2.2 Degree-level study is just like making fries …

if they are blindsided on the day of the exam board, they tend to fall back onto rules and regulations, and you will suffer as a result.

How to conduct yourself

Here is an area that is a little contradictory. On the one hand, you are a student at university and you should thoroughly enjoy your time and make the most of the experiences; at the same time, you are becoming part of a profession that expects very high standards of behavior.

For example, unlike many university courses, you will have to undergo a criminal records check, have immunization injections against hepatitis B and be expected to adhere to the CSP rules on professional conduct, etc. Just be aware that you will need to act in such a way as not to bring your profession

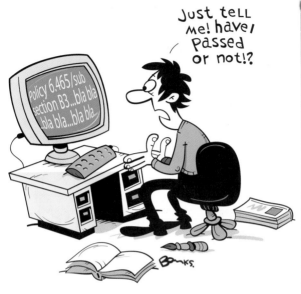

Fig. 2.3 University 'language' can be hard to digest. Just ask your tutor if you need anything interpreting!

into disrepute. It is NOT acceptable for you to skip tutorials or lectures – they are all too important and your patients deserve better.

What your lecturers expect from you

It may be useful for you to think about things from the lecturer's point of view. Here is a typical morning for me.

6am, alarm clock goes off way too soon. 6.15, I'm on the road trying to beat the traffic so I can get into the city to do some more writing up on my PhD – oh, by the way, I've also got this chapter to write. I can't remember which daughter has cheerleading, violin or netball – in fact, it may be all three at once! I've got a student coming to see me at 9 who's been in tears about her studies and her boyfriend. Supposed to go to a staff meeting but I'm double booked – shame. I've got three different topics to teach today, two of which I'm not particularly confident on. I walk into the room hoping to see an intelligent, motivated audience, instead I see this …

What would your reaction be?

Student 1 chatting to his girlfriend; after all, he does not need to concentrate, he did some anatomy on his last course. Students 2 and 3 doing each other's hair and moaning that their grant has not yet been paid in.

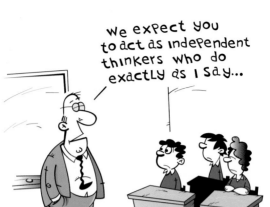

Fig. 2.4 We expect you to act as independent thinkers who do exactly as I say.

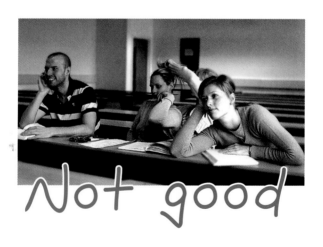

Student 4 thinking about what shoes she's going to buy tonight – her grant has gone in today. Now contrast with the picture below.

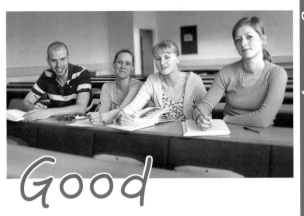

That's what I'm talking about: great eye contact, pencils at the ready, students attentive and prepared, delightful people, and I'm thinking – this is the greatest job in the world.

Now before you roll your eyes, I know it is simply not possible to act in that way every day for the entire 3 years but what I am trying to convey here is that there is no great secret to being a good student. what lecturers actually want is a basic level of human decency and manners; lecturing is a very difficult job sometimes, especially if you are relatively new to it, and it does not take much to knock the confidence of the lecturer, believe it or not, even if they appear to be brimming with confidence. Worse still (and I make no apologies for this, it's something that all human beings do in an attempt to make sense of the world), in the same way that you will form stereotypical opinions of your lecturers, we do the same about you, either individually or as a group. Trust me, you do not want to be branded as a difficult group. Stereotypes are difficult to shatter once they have been formed. So here are my tips to avoid this.

Seven steps to success

1. Turn up on time.
2. If you cannot turn up on time, at least apologize and then sit down quietly.
3. Look as though you are interested even though this may not always be the case.
4. If the lecturer asks for a volunteer, it's a very good tip to be that volunteer. Don't forget, this is the person who will be giving you a reference for your first job in 3 years' time.

5. If you have been asked to prepare some work in advance, guess what – you need to have done so.

6. Do not chew gum, send texts or have irrelevant conversations while the lecture is in progress. You would be surprised how easy it is to hear and see what a class full of students are doing – you are not hiding in the middle of a shoal of fish.

7. Once in a while, give the lecturer a compliment or at least a nice smile.

How do I get through the first year?

Below I have represented pass and failure as two mathematical formulae.

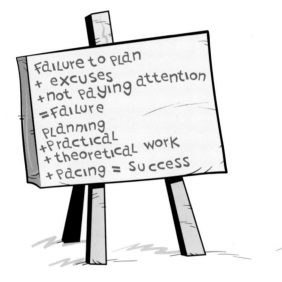

Failure to plan
+ excuses
+ not paying attention
= Failure
planning
+ practical
+ theoretical work
+ pacing = Success

What you should expect from your lecturers

The good teacher makes the poor student good and the good student superior. When our students fail, we, as teachers, too, have failed. (Marva Collins)

Contrary to what you may think, lecturers are human beings and they, like you, are all different: their likes, dislikes and expectations differ. Early on in the course, you need to work out the basic ground rules that apply for each individual lecturer.

I have always found it useful to give my students a rule sheet when I first meet them so that there is no confusion.

Ground rules

1. If you are late, come in, sit down and be quiet.
2. Turn your mobile phone off.
3. Do not use recording equipment unless by prior arrangement with the lecturer.
4. If the lecturer goes too fast or too slow, tell the lecturer; not each other.
5. Have a go, join in, relax, do your best and you will be encouraged.
6. If you miss handouts, workbooks or information. Do not expect the lecturer to repeat it just for you. It is your responsibility to catch up or get info that you missed.
7. Take part, have a go and the whole thing will be a lot more enjoyable and productive.

And now the bit you will probably read the most.

How to get through your exams

Put yourself in the lecturer's place. And by the way, you have 50 of these to mark.

Question: "Discuss how the structure of the hip joint is related to its function"

ANSWER 1

The hip joint is big and has lots of things attached to it .You know it's week if you have a trendelberg gate and you have to put you're foot down quickly. Your hip joint has menisci in between.

ANSWER 2

The knee joint is a biaxial bicondylar joint with two degrees of freedom of motion, this is necessary for its function in that it allows for the leg to rotate and lock into place when the knee is fully extended. The shape of the menisci, tension in collateral ligaments and the shape of the femoral condyles all contribute towards this.

ANSWER 3

The hip joint has a large ROM with an ASIS . # are not unusual. The PSIS is close to the NOF and treatment with PNF will prevent DVTs and PEs.

ANSWER 4

According to Jones (1911) the hip is a ball and socket joint but according to my notes it is a hinge joint.

ANSWER 5

The hip joint has a structure which is well suited to its function, the structure is a multi axial spheroidal (ball and socket) joint with three degrees of freedom of movement – these are flex/ext/abd/add/int rot/ext/rot, a combination of all these being called circumduction. The function is to take the lower limb through a large range of movement whilst retaining stability, there now follows a summary of how this is obtained. Factors contributing to mobility include the Articular cartilage, the Ball & socket shape Neck/shaft angle …

Now give each answer a mark out of 10, bearing in mind that the pass mark is 40%.

Answer 1:

Answer 2:

Answer 3:

Answer 4:

Answer 5:

Not easy, is it, and it is not over yet. Students 1, 2 and 4 are not happy with their marks. They would like some feedback from you. What do you tell them?

Why do students fail?

Let's look at the reasons why students fail or, more accurately, the reasons why students *think* they are going to fail.

1. You came into the wrong class on day one (you should have been enrolling on a Masters degree in Bulgarian Pottery) and were too scared to say anything. It's happened before –believe me!

2. You are not clever enough.

3. You party your first few months away then find that there is too much work to cram into a short time.

4. You don't like the university.

5. You think you have chosen the wrong course.

6. You suffer serious personal problems during the course.

7. You were too shy or afraid to ask for help.

8. You are abducted by aliens.

ANSWERS

1. Tell the lecturer and get to the right room before it's too late.

2. Depends on how you define "clever"; the students who do well on a tough academic degree are not always the academic geniuses. It tends to be the ones who are organized, dedicated and have a long-term strategy for their studies.

3. Not a lot we can do about this. You were probably warned about this in freshers' week; you can't do last-minute cramming on a course like physiotherapy.

4. Depends on why. It may be possible to transfer to another university but don't get your hopes up. The main thing is to be clear that it is the university that you don't like and not the subject.

5. If it is the course that you are unsure of then you must communicate with your personal tutor. You won't be letting them down and they will view this as a mature decision and you will be supported.

6. This is going to happen at some point over 3 years. Tell us – we're good but not telepathic; if we know about a problem we can usually deal with it effectively. Don't forget that your lecturers are probably physiotherapists who went into the profession because they had a desire to help people – that includes you!

7. Don't be; it takes more courage to make a fool of oneself.

8. If they are aliens with a decent knowledge of anatomy and physiology then make the most of it and return to earth just in time for your exams.

Student wisdom

As usual, my thanks go to the students without whom I would not have the job that I love and who never let me down.

"Semester 1 is really stressful, a million things go through your head and you find it hard to manage things. You feel like you aren't doing enough work. Since revising for the exams, I have found myself reading anatomy, looking at next semester's work and trying to read and research a little bit about what is to come. Even if it's only 10–20 mins of reading or looking a few things up on the computer when I'm on it a day, every little bit helps and it makes you feel more confident. Semester 1 also gives you a good idea of the rest of the course and enables you to organize and plan your workload better for semester 2." (Liz Harrison)

"The biggest concern for me when I started was the directed study and how to cope, studying in a group is the best thing ever since sliced bread! The internet connection broke in my apartment for the first semester. I realized how important it is … I had to spend most evenings in the uni." (Therese Tully)

"USE THE LIBRARY. Universities have such good facilities available for you and most of the time the books you need will be in the library so you don't have to spend hundreds of pounds buying them! (Leaves you more money to spend on shoes!) Lecturers are good at handing out reading lists and chapters which will be most relevant to you. Heed their advice, they know what they're on about.

When thing go wrong … don't panic, there is always lecturers and personal tutors willing to help, as I have learnt, they only want you to achieve the best you possibly can, don't be scared of them. It is important to work hard, but also play!

All work and no play makes physio students very boring people. It is so important that you make sure you have time to enjoy university life, explore your new surrounding city, check out the student union bar and try out all the different clubs and events that your student union lay on for you.

University is such an important time for you to discover new things: cultures, sports and yourself. But don't forget why you're there, to get your degree so play must always be carefully balanced with your workload." (Rhian Sunderland)

"I'd say is get to know some anatomy before you start. It would relieve a lot of pressure before the year begins and give you a good foundation to build the rest of the knowledge that'll be thrown at you. I'm finding learning the anatomy for the upper limb loads easier since I've already been through the experience of learning the lower limb." (Andrew Hagon)

Finally

Over the next 3 years you will make mistakes, you will do well on some things, not so well on others. You will be academically pulled, pushed and twisted, at times wondering if you are up to the challenge. All of this is normal – keep going and good luck.

Section 2
Studying physiotherapy

So then, you are in. Freshers' week is but a distant memory and now it all begins! Each physio school structure is different and subject to constant change so this is a rough guide to the core areas that you will encounter along the way. You will have a certain level of scientific understanding so remember that you are building on that foundation. If you try to leap into the meaty hard stuff that you hear on ER or Scrubs, you will drown. In the words of Kiss, "You can work real hard or just fantasize," i.e. if you want to get there, and you will get there, you just need to work at it. Physiotherapy is all about learning to walk before you run. Well, take that ethic and apply it to your learning. One thing to remember – studying a vocational degree is not like a normal academic course. You are expected to study biology, physics, biochemistry and psychology as well as manual techniques, professional practice, teaching, etc. However, it makes you an infinitely flexible individual with a broad knowledge – so all the better for it!

Chapter 3   **Anatomy and physiology** 37

Chapter 4   **Musculoskeletal physiotherapy** 45

Chapter 5   **Electrotherapy** 61

Chapter 6   **Cardiopulmonary physiotherapy** 69

Chapter 7   **Neurologic physiotherapy** 81

Chapter 8   **Pharmacology** 93

Chapter 9   **Biopsychosocial approach** 101

Chapter 10   **Pediatrics** 111

Chapter 11   **Clinical placement** 119

Anatomy and physiology
Nick Southorn

- Introduction – anatomy   38
- Introduction – physiology   41
- In the clinic   43
- Conclusion   44

Studying physiotherapy

Introduction – anatomy

It is universally accepted that anatomy is *the* subject to excel in as physiotherapists use anatomic knowledge for just about everything. Anatomy is the study of the structures of the human body, including bone, ligaments, muscles, organs, vessels and nerves. While it is often assumed that simply naming the structures is enough, it never is! As physiotherapists, you will need an exemplary knowledge of the *functional anatomy* of the human body, i.e. you will need to understand the interplay between the structures and how their shape affects their function. Once you have this knowledge, you can begin to use it therapeutically – like achieving mechanical advantage over a moment arm, utilizing anatomic features, such as the pores found in the lungs, to provide treatment and so on. Another use of anatomic knowledge comes in the form of diagnostics. The location of pain, the area of sensory loss, the limited range of movement, the palpation, the joint movement feeling, the auscultation, etc., etc., etc. You can never overestimate the importance of anatomic knowledge for the physiotherapy clinician. Ever. It is fortunate, then, that studying anatomy can be brilliant fun!

Visualizing anatomy

How you study anatomy depends on your learning style. It is helpful to make use of the university's skeleton, or buy your own, and use string, sticky tac, sticky paper and bright marker pens and get stuck in. We learn more if we are having fun so get creative and cover that skeleton!

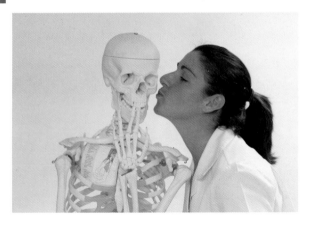

Fig. 3.1 A love of anatomy is an essential requirement for physiotherapy students.

Using this will help you visualize the structures when you are assessing your patient. Another way, if you don't have a skeleton to hand, is to use pens that are safe on human skin and color your friends in! See how creative you can get by artistically drawing the muscles and tendons or the lungs and their fields – don't forget the abdomen and the organs in there. This can be great if you celebrate Halloween and you are heading off to a party.

A great way of remembering the structures in the hand: get a pair of gloves, those yellow washing-up ones if you are feeling well off or pinch a pair of disposables from university if you aren't, and use a biro pen to write them on – you can do bones and ligaments on one hand and vessels and nerves on the other! I believe a swimming sock can do the same job for the feet. This idea has the advantage of aiding palpation skills too.

Don't forget the peripheral nerves! From what spinal segment are the muscles and skin innervated (i.e. myotomes and dermatomes)? Where are important areas of nerve bundles? Are there any areas of nerve tissue that are at particular risk of damage? This area of anatomy is easy to forget but vital for understanding a variety of conditions that affect nervous function, from fractures to swollen tissue, as well as identifying at what spinal level a problem is likely to be.

Mnemonics and chants

OK, we all know what a mnemonic is – basically making certain things easier to learn by way of chant or using the first letter of each word to create either a word or sentence. For some reason in medicine, we like to make them as grotesque as possible, which makes writing about them in a book such as this one quite challenging.

They are marvellous, though, for things that can otherwise be confused; a good mnemonic or rhyme can soon straighten things out. So here are a few of the less outrageous ones that I remember. You may wish to challenge your tutor to tell you their method of remembering certain things! They come in useful for a range of topics but we'll have a look at the anatomy ones here.

DEEP REFLEX NERVE ROOTS

One, two: buckle my shoe; three, four: kick the door; five, six: pick up the sticks; seven, eight: shut the gate.

S 1 & 2	Ankle jerk
L 3 & 4	Knee jerk
C 5 & 6	Biceps and brachioradialis
C 7 & 8	Triceps

CARPAL BONES (PROXIMAL ROW, THEN DISTAL ROW: MEDIAL TO LATERAL)

Some Lovers Try Positions That They Can't Handle.
Scaphoid
Lunate
Triquetrum
Pisiform
Trapezium
Trapezoid
Hamate

ROTATOR CUFF MUSCLES (AS THEY INSERT ONTO THE GREATER TUBERCLE OF THE HUMERUS, PROXIMAL TO DISTAL)

SITS
Supraspinatus
Infraspinatus
Teres minor
Subscapularis

BRONCHI – WHICH ONE IS MORE VERTICAL?

Inhale a *bite*; it goes down the *right*.

Small objects that are inhaled are more likely to occlude the right lung as the bronchus is more vertical.

HUMERAL FRACTURE AFFECTS:

ARM nerves (proximal to distal humerus)
Axilla (head)
Radial (midshaft)
Median (condylar)

CRANIAL NERVES IN ORDER

Oh	I	Olfactory
Once	II	Optic
One	III	Oculomotor
Takes	IV	Trochlear
The	V	Trigeminal
Anatomy	VI	Abducent
Final	VII	Facial
Very	VIII	Vestibulocochlear
Good	IX	Glossopharyngeal
Vacations	X	Vagus
Are	XI	Accessory
Heavenly	XII	Hypoglossal

ERECTOR SPINAE MUSCLES (LATERAL TO MEDIAL)

I Like Standing.
Iliocostalis
Longissimus
Spinalis

Other methods

However you do it practically, you must have concise notes to back you up. Giggling in your exams as you recall your best mate covered in paint won't help you too much! Flash cards are good for the more traditional learning style and they are easier to clean up. More and more commonly, books come with flash cards associated with them – also with interactive goodies like the "student consult" website offered by Reed Elsevier publishers on the majority of their student reference books.

Palpation is a special skill that physiotherapists need to learn. Derek Field (Field & Hutchinson 2006) has produced a particularly good palpation book. However, there are plenty to choose from. Remember that although it is helpful to read about palpation skills, nothing will replace getting hands on!

What books you buy depends on who you are. There are a range of anatomy coloring books (McCann & Wise 2008, Pinel & Edwards 2007), right through to the in-depth books of *Gray's anatomy* (Standing 2008) and Netter (2006). Whatever you get, you will need to supplement it with a solid biomechanics/ human movement book and a joint structure and function book.

Introduction – physiology

Physiology is the study of the body's tissues at a cellular level. This is an important topic which requires plenty of concentration and caffeine. Your tutors will guide you on how much depth your course demands but remember that you are to build on previous knowledge. Physiology is important as it supports our knowledge of normal human functioning. Knowing exactly how something functions is the first step to knowing how it goes wrong.

Learning physiology

This scientific subject can be dry but do your best to liven it up. Again, group work will really help here. Get a group of about four or five people and pick an organ or tissue, etc. Go away for 2 or 3 days and come back for a "teach yourself" session. Teaching is the best way to learn so you will really benefit from this. Each of you is to also write 10 questions about your topic and keep the answers safe. At the end of your teaching sessions break off into teams and have a mini pub quiz! It's a mind blowingly simple way to distract yourself from a detailed subject.

Some people like pictorial evidence of whatever it is they are learning and as such, physiology is a difficult one. However, there is a branch of physiology that allows you to see exactly what is going on and this is particularly helpful in pathophysiology. Have a look at the pictures (see next page).

In these histologic pictures you can see normal muscle tissue with and without stains compared with abnormal dystrophic muscle. It's right there – that has to be much clearer to understand than if I were to try to explain the differing fiber size, the lack of dystrophin and relate that to muscle function; you'd be rightly snoozing before long. A lovely book for this is *Human histology* (Stevens & Lowe 2004).

Warning: Only go as detailed as your course demands as you can get lost in the black hole that is physiology. Leave the ridiculously in-depth stuff to the clinical physiologists! Some good advice is look at learning physiology like you would build a house: a solid foundation is essential, i.e. get the basics to 100% before moving on. If you find that you are becoming fond of physiology then that is great news! Just make sure that you don't neglect your other subjects – you will have plenty of time after graduating to continue your study.

Some "essential" areas to be looking at are the following.

• Nerves and nerve conduction, including synapse and neuromuscular junction

• Muscle and muscle contraction

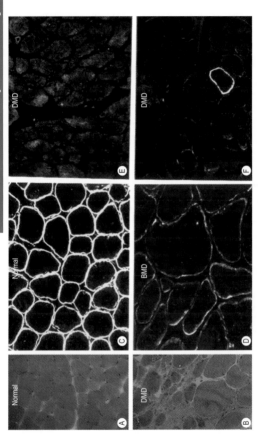

Fig. 3.2 Biopsies of normal (A, C) and dystrophic (B, D–F) muscle. C–F shows a different staining type (an antibody to dystrophin) to highlight further the differences between normal and pathologic tissue. These really show the normal structure of tissues and the physiologic effects of pathology on these tissues. (Reproduced with kind permission of Professor Caroline Sewry, Imperial College, London.)

- Pain gate theory
- Blood (specifically binding of oxygen and the dissociation curve)
- Energy cycles/production
- Cardiac function and electrical activity in the heart, vessel types and structure
- Lungs
- Bone and collagen (including tendons and ligaments)
- Renin-angiotensin cycle
- Endocrine function/regulation

These are the basics and I'm sure that your lecturers would be happy to add plenty more, such as pancreas, kidney, lymphatics, etc., but these are better learned as you experience them during placements. The advice remains the same – get the BASICS to 100% and build upon that foundation.

There is a good range of physiology books, again ranging from the coloring book to the unpalatable. Some are anatomy *and* physiology books (Martini 2006, Tortora & Derrikson 2008). These are generally very good but always ensure that the level of anatomy isn't compromised.

"Tool box"

- Hands for palpating
- Tape measure
- Goniometer (finger and standard)
- Safe-on-skin coloring pens
- An imagination!

All in all, anatomy and physiology are very practical sciences and you will occasionally feel like you are hitting your head against a wall. As long as you get the basics, the rest will all come flooding back during clinical placements, not in a "eureka" epiphany style but more of an autopilot, "where did that information come from?" kind of way.

In the clinic

During clinical placements; a good clinical educator will grill you on anatomy and physiology as they are, as previously indicated, integral to your clinical practice. On assessment, you will be considering the anatomy of the structures you are palpating, visualizing the joints moving through the range, considering what tendon runs where, from what level of the spine the innervating nerves arise, where muscles insert and originate, etc. It all forms part of your clinical reasoning. Taking a good set of notes with you is always necessary to swat up before you see a patient. The gold standard of clinical placement books is the pocket book (Kenyon & Kenyon 2009); note that the familiar pink book seen in the clutches of students since 2004 has had a funky new design for the 2009 edition.

Conclusion

You may think that I have labored the point unnecessarily regarding the importance of anatomic and physiologic knowledge. However, it really is the underpinning of our practice and should be taken seriously. Once you have all the information on board you will find that most other things fall into place. Learning about pathology is a breeze if you have a sound knowledge of anatomy and physiology and the same is true with pharmacology: if you know your physiology then you will have no problems working out what drug affects what structure and how.

References

Field, D., Hutchinson, J.O., 2006. Anatomy, Palpation and Surface Markings, fourth ed. Churchill Livingstone, Edinburgh.

Kenyon, J., Kenyon, K., 2009. The Physiotherapist's Pocket Book, second ed. Churchill Livingstone, Edinburgh.

Martini, F.H., 2006. Fundamentals of Anatomy and Physiology, seventh ed. Prentice-Hall, New Jersey.

McCann, S., Wise, E., 2008. Anatomy Coloring Book, third ed.. Kaplan Medical, California.

Netter, F.H., 2006. Atlas of Human Anatomy: Professional Edition, forth ed. Saunders, Philadelphia.

Pinel, J.P.J., Edwards, M., 2007. A Colorful Introduction to the Anatomy of the Human Brain, second ed. Pearson Educational, New Jersey.

Standing, S. (Ed.), 2008. Gray's Anatomy, fortieth ed. Churchill Livingstone, Edinburgh.

Stevens, A., Lowe, J. (Eds.), 2004. Human Histology, third ed. Edinburgh, Mosby.

Tortora, G.J., Derrikson, B., 2008. Principles of Anatomy and Physiology, twelth ed. Wiley, Chichester.

Musculoskeletal physiotherapy
Nick Southorn

- *So what is* musculoskeletal therapy?   47
- Initial subjective assessment   47
- Initial objective assessment   50
- Clinical semaphore   52
- Treatments   52
- Muscle energy techniques (MET)   55
- In the clinic   58

Studying physiotherapy

Musculoskeletal physiotherapy (MSK) is probably the largest area of physiotherapy in terms of practitioner and patient numbers. It is also the area that is common to physiotherapy around the world. MSK in this sense means orthopedic medicine, manual therapy, the alternative therapies such as osteopathy, sports medicine, Maitland, etc. Basically, MSK encompasses all the "hands on" manual techniques and exercise prescription for the relief or prevention of disorders of the musculoskeletal system. It is a culmination of detailed anatomic, physiologic, pathologic knowledge. What appears to catch most students out is the necessity of a detailed and concise assessment. As with all areas of physiotherapy, the assessment is the single most important part. The big difference here is that you are the *main* diagnostician in the treatment of *your* patient. This may mean looking at results of diagnostic imaging, blood biochemistry, nerve conduction studies, biopsies, etc, to help you develop a true clinical picture and a diagnosis.

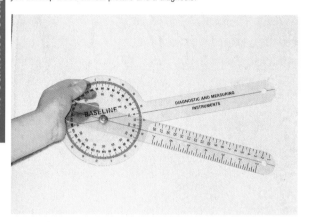

Fig. 4.1 A goniometer for precise measurements of joints is very important.

A glossary of terms may be useful to begin with: For a more comprehensive list of physiotherapy terms, *The dictionary of physiotherapy* (Porter 2005) is necessary.

- **Abduction**: movement away from the midline of the body.
- **Accessory movement**: a movement that can be done by the therapist, which makes up part of a gross overall movement. However, the patient cannot isolate and carry out this movement. For example, in shoulder abduction, the humeral head glides inferiorly in the articular surface of the glenoid cavity. A therapist can perform a passive accessory caudad glide to help improve the whole movement of abduction. The opposite is physiologic movement.
- **Active movement**: movement performed without facilitation.
- **Adduction**: movement towards the midline of the body.
- **Caudad**: movement towards the tail (literally) or towards the feet (practically).

- **Cephalic**: to do with the head (movement towards the head).
- **Extension**: a joint movement whereby the interior angle increases.
- **Flexion**: a joint movement whereby the interior angle decreases.
- **Manipulation**: high-velocity thrust moving a joint well into the limits of its range. The patient cannot stop this procedure.
- **Mobilization**: movement of a joint in such a way that the patient has total control and can stop the procedure if need be.
- **Overpressure**: the additional movement in a joint beyond the normal range that is applied by the therapist during assessment.
- **Paradigm**: a concept or belief.
- **Passive movement**: movement of a joint by the therapist.
- **Physiologic movement**: a movement of a joint such as shoulder abduction. It can be passive (i.e. no effort from the patient required as the therapist moves the joint) or active (the patient does all the work). The opposite is accessory movement.

So what is musculoskeletal therapy?

You will hear practitioners talk about the various ways in which to treat or assess a patient such as "orthopedic medicine," "McKenzie," "Maitland," "Mulligan," "Cyriax," etc. Each of these techniques has slightly different approaches and theories behind it. There are people who will vigorously stick to one particular type of treatment and there are people who "cherry pick" aspects from each. Either way, as a student physiotherapist it is essential that you consider all of them to be within your learning remit. Below is a brief taster of some of the different techniques that physiotherapists employ in their practice. It is worth noting that none of these techniques is "physiotherapy" so they are regarded as *part* of your treatment arsenal and not your only trick! As a physiotherapist, you have legal license to carry out these techniques but you may see medical doctors, osteopaths and chiropractors also using them. Of course, certain types are preferred by certain professions; osteopathy and physiotherapy are becoming more alike in their treatments as the evidence base supports treatments and the professions take them on and concentrate on them.

Initial subjective assessment

Assessments are always made up of two parts – the subjective and the objective. The former involves information gathered by questioning and the latter is what is seen and/or measured by the clinician. The initial assessment is no different but it usually involves additional information.

The clerical questions are the standard name, address, general practitioner/family physician, date of birth and so on, so that you can be sure that you have the correct patient in front of you.

Some "special questions" are typically also asked at the start. These may include queries about:

- heart or lung problems, blood pressure
- diabetes

- asthma
- rheumatoid or osteo-arthritis (be prepared to explain the difference between them)
- steroid usage
- anticoagulant therapy
- allergies
- any recent significant weight loss that can't be explained by dieting or increase in activity
- cancer.

Some questions may be guided by the type of condition, such as the cauda equina check for low back pain.

- Bladder retention/incontinence, bowel incontinence
- Saddle anesthesia
- Bilateral leg pain/weakness

Headings that may help gather a database of your patient are listed below. Something that may be of use to you is to work towards a SIN factor, which is the Severity, Irritability and Nature of the condition. While you read through these, have a think about some answers and which heading – severity, irritability or nature – they may contribute to.

PRESENTING CONDITION (PC)

- What is your *main* problem with your condition?
  - This is sometimes referred to as "question 1."
  - The information you need is: *how is this disease affecting the patient?*
  - This question will help you discover the *actual* effect on lifestyle and function as well as what the patient would like to regain.
  - You can guide the answer but try not to direct the answer: *"Is it loss of movement or strength, pain, or something else?"* or *"Is it preventing you from doing something you like or have to do?"*, etc.

HISTORY OF PRESENTING CONDITION (HPC)

- Was there a major event that led to these symptoms (like a vehicle incident) or is it a result of microtrauma (such as repetitive strain injuries)? Perhaps it just came on (insidious onset).
  - Try to gather information relating to the incident such as the mechanism of injury, were they driving or a passenger, were seatbelts worn, how far did they fall, how long before medical attention arrived, etc. Remember to be sensitive to psychologic/emotional implications relating to a major incident.
- How long have you noticed that something is not right/have you had the symptoms? Try to establish the age of the condition; is this one of many episodes or the only time this has happened?
- Did the symptoms come on immediately or develop over time?
- Are there any legal issues to consider?
- What other treatments or investigations have been used so far, if any (medical/surgical/complementary)?

LIST OF SYMPTOMS

Since you have asked about the *main* problem in question 1, they should have explained the whole story of that so now is a good time to ask what other symptoms/problems they can think of.

PAIN

- Do they have any?
- Is it constant or intermittent? Explain that constant means *all the time, 24 hours of the day.*
- Ask them to describe the pain – throbbing, sharp, dull, "toothache like," shooting, etc.
- Can they rate it out of 10? The Numerical Rating Scale (NRS) is a 0–10 scale which is very useful as an objective measure. Ask for a number between 0 and 10 to describe when the pain is at its worst, least and right now.
- Is it the same intensity or variable?
- Aggravating/easing factors – remind them that rubbing, heat and rest are valid answers here. Also explore the length of time it takes for the pain to disappear.
- Is the pain so bad sometimes that they have to miss something (like work, hobbies)?
- Diurnal pattern.
  - Do the symptoms appear worse at different times of the day (i.e. do they worsen/improve through the day or remain constant?)?
  - Sleep patterns – are they aware of the symptoms when they awaken/on rising from bed/through the night (does it wake them)? If so, how many hours of unbroken sleep do they get?

PAST MEDICAL AND SURGICAL HISTORY (PMH)

Simply a list of conditions and operations that the patient has had in the recent past. Some things may appear insignificant to the pathology you face, such as the patient with adhesive capsulitis who tells you that they also have hypothyroidism or diabetes mellitus – the two have been likened to adhesive capsulitis (Siegel et al 1999).

DRUG HISTORY (DH)

Just a list of medication they take plus any other drugs they may wish to inform you of. Remind the patient that it is not only prescribed medications you need to be aware of – many people will buy their own from a pharmacy or herbalist.

SOCIAL HISTORY (SH)

- What do they do for a living?
  - Has this condition had an impact on their job?
  - Is it possible that their job may have caused this condition? Be *very* careful not to imply or let them infer that their employer is to blame for their discomfort.

- Hobbies
  - Is this condition preventing them from pursuing their hobbies?
  - Is it possible that their hobby has contributed to the condition?
- Home circumstances.
  - Can they carry out activities of daily living (ADL)? Personal ADLs (PADLs) include washing, dressing, brushing teeth, etc. Domestic ADLs (DADLs) include cleaning, cooking, driving, etc. Establishing this will give you an indication not only about their ability to function but also their dependency on other people. This can be quite an emotive topic as sometimes it is quite humbling to have lost a certain degree of independence.
  - Who do they live with? Do they have dependants? Is the person they have become dependent on capable of coping with this new situation?
  - Do they have stairs and can they negotiate the stairs *safely*?

So there it is – the basic checklist of subjective questioning that will create for you a comprehensive database of the patient. Having asked these questions, you will have a good idea of the SIN factor, the patient's motivation for recovery, the patient's priorities, and the gross effect of this condition.

Initial objective assessment

The objective assessment is the method by which you discover the clinical signs of the pathology rather than just the symptoms. It is good practice to obtain information from the other side too and comment on whether anything you find (such as swelling) is of long standing or a new sign. As with the subjective assessment, it is always helpful to have a system in place. A detailed assessment is a thorough one that extends way beyond the realms of joint measurements. As a medical professional, you should note any other significant observations. Below is a brief guide to the objective assessment.

OBSERVATIONS

- Bulk.
  - As this is objective, you should get a measurement of swelling. In doing so, you will also note the placement of the tape measure (e.g. L ankle circumference 30 cm measured at 2 cm above lateral malleolus). It is also worth measuring the opposite side for comparison.
  - Muscle atrophy/hypertrophy – again, you can get a tape measure around it.
- Skin color.
- Condition of skin and nails.
  - Dry skin
  - Abrasions, ulcers, etc.
  - Brittle nails
  - Abnormal hair growth
  - Other abnormal growths

- Artefacts.
  - Any walking aids, braces, orthotics, catheter, bandages, etc. in situ?
  - How well do they fit? Any red markings, etc? Appropriate use of stick/frame?

POSTURE

- Standing and sitting posture.
  - Are they symmetric (folds/shoulders creases, etc.)?
  - Do they have a kyphotic (excessive thoracic curve), lordotic (excessive lumbar curve), lateral shift (shoulders not aligned with hips, usually indication of disk herniation or facet joint irritation) or flat back (no curve) posture?
  - Any scoliosis (lateral spinal curvature)?
  - Do they lean and prop to one side?
  - Do they become uncomfortable quickly?
  - Do they have a good base of support?
  - Is there rotation at the hips?
  - Are the feet excessively turned in or out?
  - Is one knee bent in standing?

GAIT

- What are the feet doing?
  - Heel strike
  - Follow through – as the foot becomes flat on the ground, does it roll out to the side or into the middle (pronate or supinate)?
  - Toe off – is dorsiflexion achieved or did they compensate?
  - Swing phase – do the toes clear the ground satisfactorily?
  - Are they facing the direction of travel
- What are the hips doing?
  - Are the hips level through the gait cycle or do they bob up and down (Trendelenburg gait)?
  - Are they rotating at all?
- What is the upper body doing?
  - Are the arms swinging?
  - Is the body rotating normally?
  - What does the patient's face look like – are they in pain?

RANGE OF MOVEMENT (ROM)

- Measure the joints above and below the pathologic one.
  - Passive and active
  - Quality of movement
  - What is the limiting factor? Pain/stiffness, etc.
- Are you aware of the normal joint ranges?
- Use of the goniometer is essential for accuracy. Remember – left and right!

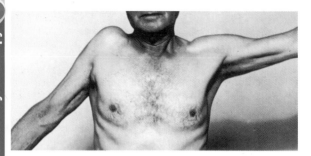

Fig. 4.2 This reverse scapulohumeral rhythm is obvious but not all conditions of movement are as easy to spot. (Reproduced from Magee 2008, with kind permission from Elsevier.).

- Functional or gross movement.
  - Rather than just checking simple flexion of the elbow, ask the patient to scratch their ear or touch their nose to see how the limb works as a unit.
  - For backs, forward flexion, side flexion, rotation and extension need to be observed.

Clinical semaphore

Any healthcare practitioner needs to know the signs and symptoms that should ring alarm bells. Currently, a common system is the red and yellow flags.

Red flags are physical risk factors that require co-ordinated care from the patient's general practitioner or, in some cases, immediate referral to the emergency department. Red flags include (nonexhaustive list): considerable unexplained weight loss, unremitting night pain, cauda equina symptoms (bladder and bowel incontinence or retention, saddle anesthesia), pulsatile mass in the abdomen, progressive motor/sensory loss in lower limbs, etc.

Yellow flags are psychologic risk factors that may hinder the treatment and hence recovery and can include (nonexhaustive list): inappropriate thoughts regarding condition, i.e. pain = harm, catastrophizing, a substantial amount of time off work, excessive visits to health professionals recently, depression, and so on.

A whole system of flags is in use, including black (work conditions that may inhibit rehab), blue (perception of work) and orange (significant psychologic issues, including drug abuse). Not all clinicians subscribe to this method so even if you become the oracle of flags you should check local policy for abbreviations in clinical notes before you use them.

Treatments

The treatments in musculoskeletal therapy vary, as previously mentioned. Rather than explain the individual treatment techniques, I have given a brief description of the treatment concepts and general information relating to some of the less obvious treatments.

Maitland

Detailed information regarding Maitland treatments can be found in probably the two most important books for Maitland practitioners: *Maitland's peripheral manipulation* (Hengeveld & Banks 2005) and *Maitland's vertebral manipulation* (Maitland et al 2005). Geoff Maitland is an Australian physiotherapist who revolutionized the teaching of vertebral manipulations and the approach of adapting techniques for neuromusculoskeletal conditions. A thorough assessment including not only the joint *ranges* but also the movement *quality* is key for Maitland practitioners.

The themes that a physiotherapist should use to approach a patient are as follows (Hengeveld & Banks 2005).

- The patient-centered approach to dealing with movement disorders. This is a commitment to the patient in terms of concentration, revisiting the information given to you by the patient until it makes sense, being nonjudgmental, having a skilled understanding of all types of communication, and understanding the science of the condition (i.e. what a clinician should know).

- The brick wall approach and the primacy of clinical evidence. This is making a distinction between the theory and diagnosis of a condition and the clinical history (i.e. the two are on either side of a permeable brick wall). This will allow the clinician to separate the signs and symptoms (the clinical) from the science (the theory), fostering a treatment that is guided by the patient's condition rather than by a "diagnosis." The message is – treat the symptoms, not the diagnosis.

- The paradigm of identifying and maximizing movement potential. This is quite self-explanatory.

- The science and art of assessment. This too is quite self-explanatory, except you need to remember that assessments are ongoing, not just something you do when you first meet a patient.

The techniques are fairly simple to understand (you will need to learn the physiology of why they work, however). The main reasons for mobilization are pain and range. The "grades" used in Maitland underpin these reasons.

- Grade I – small-amplitude movement without resistance (i.e. you don't move far and don't enter into the range of the joint).

- Grade II – large-amplitude movement with small amounts of resistance.

- Grade III – large amplitude into range.

- Grade IV – small amplitude in range (i.e. not a great deal of movement but right at the end of the joint range.

It won't take a lot of effort to grasp the idea that the lower grades are aimed at pain and the higher grades are aimed at range of movement. Do you know *why*? One thing to always consider is: how much can the patient tolerate? Maybe you will have to start with a lower grade to lower the pain levels before you take the joint into range.

- Grade V – this is a manipulation rather than a mobilization.

Cyriax/orthopedic medicine

Further information relating to Cyriax and orthopedic medicine can be found on the website of the Society of Orthopedic Medicine (SOM): www.somed.org. James Cyriax was a physician who noticed that there were, at the time, many undiagnosed and poorly treated conditions affecting the musculoskeletal system. He set about developing a system of assessment and diagnosis for these as well as nonsurgical treatments for soft tissue lesions (SOM 2004).

The principles of Dr Cyriax and therefore orthopedic medicine were:

• all pain has a source

• all treatment must reach the source

• all treatment must benefit the lesion.

We now know that pain is much more complex than this (see Professor Paul Watson's contribution, Chapter 9) and thus orthopedic medicine has undergone constant development and reappraisal in light of evidence.

Examination by tissue tension is a pillar of the Cyriax concept too. The idea is simple – if a tissue is damaged, it will be painful to pull. Dr Cyriax devised three principles to back this.

• Isometric contractions test the function of the contractile tissues.

• Passive movements test the function of the inert structures.

• The capsular pattern differentiates between joint conditions and other structural lesions.

It is for these reasons that physiotherapists trained in orthopedic medicine are hot on their functional anatomy as the concept deals with identifying the slightest imbalance or irregularity and the structure involved. The treatments involve mobilizations and soft tissue massage together with electrotherapeutic agents.

McKenzie

Robin McKenzie is not only a lucky chap but also a very astute physiotherapist from New Zealand. Legend has it that, while treating a back patient with little success, Robin told him to lie down on the plinth while he got ready. Robin walked in to find his patient lying prone (on his front) but with the head break in the bed so that the patient was in extreme back extension. The patient explained that this was the most comfortable position for him as it reduced the pain in his back. A lesser physiotherapist may have dismissed such a comment (well, they would have done in the mid 1950s, which is when this story is said to have happened). However, Robin formed a spinal treatment from it that is widely used by physiotherapists and orthopedic surgeons today. The idea is to "centralize the pain" by exercises. It is postulated that in a posterior disk hernia, an extension will express pressure over the posterior aspect of the disk, forcing the gelatinous nucleus pulposus back into a central position. This will provide pain relief, allowing more effective exercise to be carried out. A true McKenzie practitioner will not use other modalities in practice such as acupuncture or heat.

Acupuncture

Acupuncture is administered by trained physiotherapists for the relief of pain and relaxation. It has been in use for over 3000 years in the Far East, a method that has really stood the test of time. Two theories are used: the Traditional Chinese Medicine (TCM) approach and the Western medicine approach. As medical practitioners, it is important to ensure that the aspects of acupuncture with a sturdier scientific base are delivered, and the use of other aspects is not justifiable until they have similar backing. As it stands, pain management is the only indication for acupuncture in the UK.

The ancient Chinese believed that the body's health is dependent on the smooth and balanced movement of qi (energy) through meridians (channels). A number of factors can affect the flow, including the weather, stress, fear, infection, etc. The insertion of needles in the right places can free the flow, stimulating the body's own healing power.

The Western approach has the benefit of modern investigations such as functional magnetic resonance imaging (fMRI). However, there are many questions that remain unanswered by Western science and many theories that are yet to be proven. Without wanting to get carried away, here is just one development in the search for an answer to a 3000-year-old question. A recent study (Dhond et al 2008) showed increased connectivity in many parts of the brain during and after acupuncture, in particular the anterior cingulate cortex (ACC), which is known to be involved in the downregulation of pain (the way pain perception is controlled by the brain). However, although evidence would appear to support the use of acupuncture for pain, we don't know the exact consequences of the increased activity in the ACC. It is therefore hard to make a solid link between the reduction of perceived pain and the increased activity in the ACC during acupuncture. The pain gate theory is also used for acupuncture, stimulation of mechanoreceptors "closing the gate." Simple relaxation is another theory; we know that when you are more relaxed, the pain you feel is reduced.

I will not go any further but I advise you to speak to a practicing physiotherapist who uses acupuncture. I am sure that they would love to discuss the theories and science behind it all.

Muscle energy techniques (MET)

This technique is commonly used by osteopaths and physiotherapists and is based on the fact that to increase a joint range, it is necessary to overcome the neuromuscular barrier (i.e. the reflex contraction following stimulation of the Golgi body). The principle is that this reflex arc will fatigue with excessive use and can therefore be overcome. There are a few techniques to learn.

Reciprocal inhibition is simply the fact that contraction of an agonist will exert an inhibitory effect upon the contraction of its antagonist. Let's think about the elbow – during biceps contraction (the agonist), the triceps (its antagonist) will relax and allow additional force to be expressed over it (i.e. a stretch).

Postisometric relaxation works by the principle that maximal contraction is followed by maximal relaxation. The reflex arc will enter a phase of refraction and thus will tolerate a stretch being applied without activation of the muscle.

Sustained stretch is arguably a MET but is simply the sustained stretch over a muscle that will eventually fatigue the reflex arc and allow greater range to be achieved.

MULLIGAN

Brian Mulligan is a New Zealand physiotherapist who cites McKenzie, Maitland and Cyriax as being influential in his development of this system of manual therapy. The concept relates to traditional physiotherapy at its best. The idea is that the therapist should provide a sustained parallel or perpendicular glide to a joint to the end of range pain free to increase the overall range of movement. There are two types of movement considered by the concept.

- Sustained natural apophyseal glides (SNAG) – a vertebral mobilization.

- Mobilization with movement (MWM) – a passive accessory movement with active (or passive) physiologic movement of the joint.

The Mulligan concept can be easily used in conjunction with any of the above as an adjunct or as a stand-alone treatment option. It is easily carried out by the therapist and can even be taught to the patient with relative ease.

Myofascial therapy

The nice thing about myofascial therapy is that it has had a multiprofessional evolution through the years. In the 1920s German physiotherapists used Bindegewebsmassage (connective tissue massage) and osteopaths of the time used a technique that later became known as the "fascial twist." The technique progressed further with an American medical doctor called Janet Travell in the 1940s. Dr Travell first used the terminology we use today – trigger point and myofascial therapy. The technique is still used today by these three professions with great effect.

The myofascia is connective tissue that can become adhered to surrounding tissues following injury, inflammation, poor posture, etc., resulting in inhibited movement and pain. The technique is simply a soft tissue manipulation that releases the myofascia, allowing normal healing to occur. Onlookers will see the practitioner enthusiastically driving an elbow into their patient's body; this is because considerable force is sometimes needed for deeper tissues.

Pilates

Developed by Joseph Pilates as a method of rehabilitation for German soldiers returning from the Great War, this concept is based on the control and co-ordination of the muscles, especially core muscles controlling the torso and spinal column. Pilates is an excellent adjunct to the more traditional physiotherapy techniques for all types of patients as it not only encourages better core stability, it empowers the patient, making them the locus of control over their condition, and that is probably the most effective treatment you can give.

Pilates was once delivered by way of a machine called a "reformer" but now it is essentially a form of mat work exercise that allows certain postural positions to be practiced and enhanced. The idea is that all movements are purposeful and controlled. The original theory also encompassed breathing techniques to purge the body of toxins and deliver high quantities of oxygen to the tissues.

Many physiotherapists are now completing "clinical Pilates" courses which allow them to safely teach the techniques as a therapeutic exercise specific to the patient's pathology.

Exercise therapy

Therapeutic exercise is defined as the systematic and planned performance of bodily movements, postures or physical activity to remediate or prevent injury, restore or improve physical function, reduce health-related risk factors, and optimize overall health (Kinser & Colby 2002). Exercise is one of the earliest forms of physiotherapy treatment. Physiotherapists are renowned for their knowledge of therapeutic exercise and it remains one of the most common treatments used. One of the reasons is similar to that for Pilates treatments – the patient achieves a sense of ownership over their rehabilitation. This is a double-edged idea, however: if your patient lacks motivation, do you think they will do the home exercises? The answer, alas, is no! For this reason, part of the skill of prescribing home exercise is placing the emphasis on them that is appropriate for the patient. If the patient is ultra motivated and willing then a large portion of the therapy can be home exercise. If not, then you give some home exercises and make more effort in the clinic.

Learning about exercise isn't just a matter of thinking "Well, he has weak biceps, I'll give him some biceps curls." There are many things to consider.

- Am I trying to achieve increased strength or stamina? How does that influence the prescription?
- Can the patient achieve contraction against gravity? What do you do if they cannot?
- How many repetitions (number of times they lift the weight) and sets (number of times they are to perform all the repetitions)?
- How much weight do I use?
- How long should a stretch be applied for?

Sometimes you will be inclined to give general exercise advice for someone who is looking to improve general fitness and maybe lose weight. This is within the scope of the physiotherapist and something that you should relish the opportunity to do. As with all types of exercise prescription, you should consider the following.

- *Warm-up* – this is vital. Do not forget to give appropriate advice relating to an effective but not exhausting warm-up.
- *Environment* – this has to be nondistracting and conducive to exercise but above all **SAFE**.
- *Amount to do* – this is easily worked out. You must *always* ask the patient to carry out the exercises you are giving them and, in some cases, show them. Time how long it takes for them to carry out these tasks and decide whether or not you have given too much. You may think that you are doing them a service by giving them 2 hours' worth of workout but realistically, who is going to stick to that?
- *Pain* – another reason why you get them to demonstrate the exercises. If it is painful, you will have to redesign the workout.
- *Times of the day* – when do you suggest they do this? Largely, it is considered counterproductive to get someone doing hard physical activity 2 hours before going to bed as they may be aching and lose sleep.

- *Are they compensating?* Again, watch the patient as they give you a demonstration! Even in good health, you will see people cheating at exercise. I do it all the time and I am quite sure most of you do at some point too! Next time you go to the gym, watch the big macho man doing biceps curls: how much of that action is elbow flexion and how much is back extension followed by additional flexion once he has overcome the gravity line? Also, how fast do some people do leg presses? That is simply using momentum to your advantage, i.e. cheating!

  Patients are amazing at compensating – you will never tire of spotting their very subtle ways to overcome gravity or recruit other muscles to take over.

All in all, therapeutic exercise is something that you should spend a great deal of time studying regardless of the clinical area you head towards. Two excellent books for understanding exercise are *Therapeutic exercise: foundations and techniques* (Kisner & Colby 2002) and *Therapeutic exercise for lumbopelvic stabilization* (Richardson et al 2004).

Massage

Massage is something that is often confused in physiotherapy; there is a difference between the massage you get with a masseur and the therapeutic massage you will provide as a physiotherapist. I don't envy the female physiotherapists who have to put up with the moronic sleaze bag claiming "I have a groin strain injury – can I have a massage?" If they knew that you are far more likely to get hands on with some serious deep transverse friction massage than a nice soothing rub down, perhaps they would forget it.

Having said that, with your anatomic knowledge and understanding of the physiologic effects of massage, there is no reason why you can't use "normal" massage for therapeutic relaxation.

A good definition of massage is provided by Holey & Cook (1997):

Massage is the manipulation of the soft tissues of the body by a trained therapist as a component of a holistic therapeutic intervention. (p3)

A well-conducted therapeutic massage can:

- promote flow of bodily fluids (lymphatic, edematous, blood, etc.)
- reduce muscle soreness and spasm
- reduce pain in general
- mobilize connective tissue
- promote normal remodeling of tissues
- promote the release of endorphins.

The deep transverse friction massage mentioned earlier is a deep manipulation of specific tissues and can relieve pain, improve function and increase blood flow to the area, kick starting the inflammatory processes. This is a skilled massage and involves a detailed anatomic knowledge as getting it wrong will be hellishly uncomfortable for the patient.

In the clinic

As you can see, there is an awful lot that falls under the heading of musculoskeletal physiotherapy. During your placement, however, you will find that if you have a good underlying knowledge of anatomy, physiology and pathophysiology, it all falls into place quite nicely. It is always useful to have an aide mémoire for anatomy and pathology in your pocket but it is essential to have a book that details objective assessments in orthopedics because there are so many.

I have only scratched the surface of this diverse and challenging topic but I hope you will feel that you know a little more about the practice of orthopedic/musculoskeletal medicine.

References

Dhond, R.P., Yeh, C., Park, K., Kettner, N., Napadow, V., 2008. Acupuncture Modulates Resting State Connectivity in Default and Sensorimotor Brain Networks. Pain 136, 407–418.

Hengeveld, E., Banks, K., 2005. Maitland's Peripheral Manipulation, Fifth ed. Butterworth-Heinemann, Edinburgh.

Holey, E., Cook, E., 1997. Therapeutic Massage. WB Saunders, London.

Kisner, C., Colby, L.A., 2002. Therapeutic Exercise: Foundations and Techniques, Fourth ed. F A Davis, Philadelphia.

Magee, D.J., 2008. Orthopedic Physical Assessment, Fifth ed. Saunders, Philadelphia.

Maitland, G., Hengeveld, E., Banks, K., English, K., 2005. Maitland's Vertebral Manipulation. Butterworth-Heinemann, Oxford.

Porter, S., 2005. Dictionary of Physiotherapy. Butterworth-Heinemann, Edinburgh.

Richardson, C., Hodges, P., Hides, J., 2004. Therapeutic Exercise For Lumbopelvic Stabilization: A Motor Control Approach For the Treatment and Prevention Of Low Back Pain, Second ed. Churchill Livingstone, Edinburgh.

Siegel LB, Cohen NJ, Gall EP 1999 Adhesive capsulitis: a sticky issue. American Family Physician. Available at: www.aafp.org/afp/990401ap/1843.html.

Society of Orthopedic Medicine (SOM) 2004 About orthopedic medicine. Available at: www.somed.org/about.htm.

5

Electrotherapy
Tim Watson

- What is it?   62
- Why is it important?   64
- Useful ways to study   64
- Resources and information   65

Studying physiotherapy

What is it?

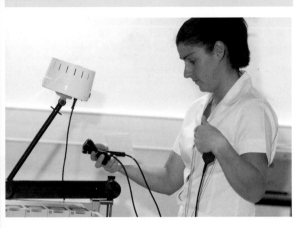

Fig. 5.1 Don't worry, electrotherapy is not all wires and plug sockets.

Electrotherapy has been a core component of physiotherapy practice since the very early days of the profession. The whole of electrotherapy goes in and out of fashion and within electrotherapy, different modalities continue to go in and out of fashion on an alarmingly regular basis which doesn't help when trying to get to grips with it as a subject.

The term "electrotherapy" is not actually very well suited for the context in which it is used. Strictly speaking, electrotherapy relates specifically to the use of electric currents to either treat disease or stimulate nerves and muscles. Within physiotherapy practice, the term "electrotherapy" is taken to include a wide range of treatment modalities (ultrasound, laser, pulsed shortwave, etc.) in addition to the use of electric currents. There is a move towards a change in the general term and electrophysical agents (EPA) is probably the better one to use and is likely to become the norm in the next few years. I will use the term electrotherapy here in its widest context, not just in terms of electric current treatments.

OK, so what *is* electrotherapy and why do physios use it at all? Well, it is a useful part of the treatment toolkit; it is a means of getting the body to respond to a stimulus in much the same way as it responds to a manual therapy stimulus or an exercise-based stimulus. The only real difference is that in electrotherapy, the stimulus comes from a machine, whether TENS, ultrasound, laser, interferential or myriad others.

It is important to realize that electrotherapy does not belong to physios – there are many other medical and allied professionals who employ electrotherapy in their practice. Historically, we might have been the most avid users within the health service, but it certainly is not something that is exclusive to us.

All electrotherapy works on a pretty straightforward basis, and I will include a very brief version of it here. A fuller explanation can be found in Watson (2008) or on the electrotherapy.org website.

The model is that you apply some energy from a machine, the effect of which is to cause a change in physiologic behavior in the tissues, and we use this change in behavior to bring about a therapeutic benefit. Working in the clinical environment, the best thing is to use the same model but turn it around and work through it in what appears to be a reverse direction. Start with the patient and their problem(s). Decide what you want to achieve and then step back through the model and decide which physiologic response you need in order to get the result you are looking for.

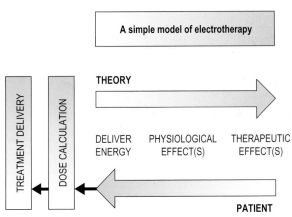

A simple model of electrotherapy

Fig. 5.2 A simple model of electrotherapy.

Having determined the bit of physiology you need to activate, come back through the model again, and decide which *modality* is most able to help, based on the available evidence. If there is not a modality that does the job you need then electrotherapy is not appropriate for this patient at the moment (though that might change as their clinical status shifts). Having chosen the best modality for the job, the next thing is to determine the *dose* of energy that will be necessary and then the last step is to "apply" the treatment.

The effects of electrotherapy are both modality and dose dependent. Get them both right and you can expect a positive outcome. Get one or the other wrong and you will not achieve the optimal result. This is no different from manual therapy, exercise therapy, acupuncture, drug therapy or any other intervention in medicine.

Electrotherapy is simply another way to trigger a physiologic response in the tissues. There is a lot of detail that one could add here, but this basic principle is the best one to hang on to in order to understand what we are trying to do. It is rarely best used in isolation – the integration of electrotherapy with other interventions is almost always the optimum way forward. It is not "magic" and is no more clever or important than anything else in the treatment toolkit, but it is a useful additional type of intervention when employed effectively.

I have described the basic mechanism of action using a physiologic intervention model. A lot of people talk about the "placebo" effect of electrotherapy, and some practitioners suggest that all electrotherapy is based on placebo. Well, I would suggest from the evidence that this is clearly not true, but I fully acknowledge that *some* of the effects of electrotherapy are placebo related (as are some bits of acupuncture, manipulation and exercise – nothing new there). In short, anybody who dismisses electrotherapy on the basis that it is all placebo has not studied the evidence.

There are as many different ways of classifying electrotherapy modalities as there are authors, I reckon. No one classification system is "right" and whichever system is used leaves a gap somewhere or another. By all means have a look at the classification and terminologies proffered in other books, but don't get too hung up about learning them as they are in a constant state of flux as "new modalities" come along and make the groupings fail one way or another. There is an international group working at the moment on coming up with an electrotherapy classification and terminology system that will be acceptable to all therapists in all countries (dream on!) but until then, the existing groupings provide a useful guide.

Why is it important?

Despite the current trend for electrotherapy to be out of fashion, it *is* important because it offers the therapist a range of tools to get better treatment out-comes with patients. Therapists who never use electrotherapy are almost certainly denying their patient some useful therapy. Practitioners who use it for everything are probably not making the best treatment choice based on the available evidence.

When used at the right place at the right time for the right reason (and at the right dose, of course), it has a phenomenal capacity to do good. Used at the wrong place and the wrong time for the wrong reason, it is just as useless as any treatment used in this way.

There is a very substantial evidence base that identifies what each electrotherapy modality is good for and what it cannot achieve. Some therapists discount electrotherapy as something for which there is no evidence but this really is not true. If you just took one modality, TENS for example, it would not be difficult to find several thousand references in the published literature that identify what it does, what it does not do, and when it is best used. Clearly, it is difficult as a student to read through several thousand papers for each and every intervention. The key is to start with the most general material and work your way through to the more specific as you need to (see next section). The point is that there *is* a substantial evidence base and even if you can't access it all and read every paper, there are people out there who have, so in the first instance, it might be a good idea to see what they have to say about it and work from there.

Useful ways to study

One of the hardest things about electrotherapy, and something that puts a lot of people off, is when you start from the physics (not usually a popular combination with physio!). Although electrotherapy is based on both physics and physiology principles, it is better to get the idea of what a modality is first, see what it is supposed to be able to do and when to use it, and then come back to the detail. The hardest thing is to start with the detail and work through to the clinical applications. I know that a lot of purists start with the formulas, numbers and equations, but I reckon that puts off more people than it turns on! Get to grips with what the modality is (and what it is not) before worrying about the detail. Use a textbook introduction or review paper, then move on to specific research papers if they help. Get the *overview* before attempting the *detail* (this is not something that only applies to undergrads – I work the same way even if I am talking to therapists who have been qualified for a while and are trying to get to grips with a new modality).

Journal reviews can be of value; they are often put together by researchers or research students and will be more up to date than textbooks. However, the texts will provide useful background and probably make the best starting point. Don't assume that all papers, reviews and texts are right; some people, with the best will in the world, make mistakes or change their mind as new evidence comes along. I know I have changed my mind on several things over the years so keep your mind open and flexible.

Anecdotal evidence (when clinicians have found something to be useful) remains of value, and just because something has not been published does not mean that it is useless or not worth serious consideration. There are lots of things in physio which appear to work, but for which there is no "hard" evidence yet. This is not an excuse for trying to justify treatments without doing research; there are simply not enough people out there doing and publishing research to cover all the bases – true in electrotherapy, just as it is for other areas of therapy.

As a general guide, when trying to find out about a modality or treatment, I would suggest that you start with the general texts (see below) and move from there to the more detailed material. It is much easier than trying to get to grips with the detail of some research project, only to find that not having a grasp of the basics makes it almost incomprehensible.

The other thing to bear in mind is that there are contraindications to all electrotherapy modalities. They might just seem like long lists when you first come across them, but they are important. You should be mindful of which contraindications might apply to your patient before you launch into a treatment. It is not a nice feeling to get halfway through something and then realize that you really should not be doing X or Y. There is nothing wrong with checking the contraindications if you are not sure, certainly better than guessing or hoping. There are lists and tables of the main ones that are easily accessible, so grab a copy of a quickie guide and keep it handy.

Resources and information

There is a wide range of sources of information related to electrotherapy. Some are easy to access and others will take a bit of searching out. Remember that electrotherapy does not belong to physiotherapy and therefore sources from other areas (e.g. physiology, sports science, psychology) might provide information in addition to publications relating to other professional groups (e.g. nursing, osteopathy, podiatry, various complementary therapies).

It is important to remember that some sources of information (books, manufacturer's booklets, web pages) may have a vested interest in trying to convince you of one view or another or to try and sell you something. It is often difficult to establish who has written some of this material and on what it is based. There is no problem accessing it – you are encouraged to do so – but you need to retain a healthy skepticism as you would with information in any other area.

WEB

There are lots of things related to electrotherapy on the Web. Some are great and informative and accurate. Others are dire, completely untrue and simply trying to get money from people. If you are not sure who has written something, be skeptical. Even if you do think you know who has done the writing, still be skeptical. Remember that anybody can publish just about anything on a web page. It does not have to be true or accurate or meaningful. Clearly one would hope that people would not deliberately try and mislead you, but it happens (not just in electrotherapy).

The website that I run (www.electrotherapy.org) is independent (not trying to sell anything) and is updated as the evidence changes. It is free, open access and you can download whatever you want, though please do acknowledge where it has come from. There are also links to many other sites and resources which you might find useful.

BOOKS

There are a lot of books around on electrotherapy. Some are general texts and some are very specific. Some are great and some contain info that is incorrect, out of date or providing a very skewed view. Two recent texts will provide general info that might help you while a student.

- Robertson V, Ward A, Low J, Reed A 2007 Electrotherapy explained. Elsevier, Edinburgh. This is a good general text which covers all the essentials including background, research evidence and clinical application. Worth having a copy or making sure that you have access to it. There are copies in many departments, but be careful to look at the latest edition as things have changed quite a lot from the previous editions.

- Watson T 2008 Electrotherapy: Evidence Based Practice. Elsevier, Edinburgh. This is edited by Tim Watson and also published by Elsevier in 2008. It is not designed as a "how to do it" text but, as the title implies, it does set out the evidence for each modality. Each chapter is written by an expert in their field, and it is about as up to date as you can get in terms of evidence review in a text.

I also did a chapter on electrotherapy in the latest edition of Tidy's physiotherapy (S Porter, Elsevier 2008) and while it cannot possibly cover the detail, it does give a general introduction to each of the common modalities – might be useful for the overview stuff.

There are numerous other texts around, reviewed and listed on the website (www.electrotherapy.org), should you want to look at alternatives.

ARTICLES

As mentioned, there are many journal articles that look at specific issues and research in electrotherapy. These are fantastically useful when you are looking for the detail and current evidence but they are often a bit heavy as a starting point. Do remember that there are journals that publish reviews rather than detailed research papers, and these provide an invaluable resource when you are trying to get to grips with what the current story is. Remember that a textbook will have been written a while before it actually reaches the shelf and things will have changed between the writing and you reading it. While reviews in journals still go out of date, they are often more up to date than a text from a few years back. *Physical Therapy Reviews* is a journal dedicated to review papers while others publish useful reviews now and then, including: *Physiotherapy Research International, Advances in Physiotherapy, Physical Therapy in Sport, Manual Therapy* and *Physiotherapy Theory and Practice*.

NEWSLETTERS

There are a couple of newsletters out there that give a commentary on recent research. I do an Electrotherapy Newsletter every 2–3 months and try to include all the research which I have found in that time together with a summary of the paper and a commentary on what it might mean in terms of practice. Access is free and you can register by email from the www. electrotherapy.org website.

CSP PUBLICATION(S)

The Chartered Society of Physiotherapy (in the UK) has a couple of publications that are worth looking out for, especially the 2006 *Guidance for the clinical use of electrophysical agents* (2006) which includes contraindications and practice issues. Some departments will have a copy (I think that they should have) but if not, you will almost certainly find a copy in your university library.

MANUFACTURER'S HANDBOOKS AND INFORMATION

All machines come with a handbook. Some are great and are not especially wonderful but at the very least, they do identify what each button, switch and dial on the machine does, which can be a good starting point even if nobody in the department knows what they do (I am afraid to say that it does happen like that sometimes). Some of the handbooks go a lot further and give some additional information about treatments and uses, but remember that the manufacturers do not always provide copious evidence to back up their claims so once again, be constructively critical about what you read.

In addition to specific machine handbooks, several manufacturers produce more general booklets about electrotherapy modalities or treatment programs which are worth a look if you can get hold of them. The reps from the electrotherapy companies do visit departments now and then, and it is always worth having a chat to them to see what they have (other than pens and freebie goniometers!).

Top tips

- Don't be put off by the physics or complex terminology.
- Get the big picture before you start worrying about the detail.
- Look at general texts first, then the more detailed and specific stuff after that.

- Consider the integration of electrotherapy with other interventions – it is rarely best when applied in isolation.
- Do know the critical contraindications.
- Don't be afraid to ask how a machine operates if you are not sure or find the handbook if nobody seems to know.
- Beware of anybody who dismisses all electrotherapy as useless or, for that matter, anybody who claims it is the answer to everything!
- Do be critical of the evidence and challenge the claims made; that is how we all make progress.

Student Wisdom

"While using electrotherapy on placements, make sure you understand how to use that particular model *before* you need it! There is nothing more embarrassing than tentatively and unconfidently searching for the 'on' button!

Always have a 'lay' explanation for your patients as to the nature of the treatment you are about to provide. This will allow them to relate to the treatment better – but also be prepared to give a well-structured explanation too. There is always the possibility that your patient has a reasonable understanding already." (Mark Bowe, Manchester)

Reference

Watson, T., 2008. Electrotherapy: Evidence Based Practice. Elsevier, Edinburgh.

6

Cardiopulmonary physiotherapy
Mandy Jones

- Learning the theory   70
- Preparation for clinical placement   73
- Conclusion   79

Studying physiotherapy

So here it is, the Marmite of physiotherapy! Students tend to either love or hate this clinical area, with little opinion in between. The fact that physiotherapists even work with patients with cardiopulmonary problems often comes as a surprise, and it's not uncommon to hear students say "Respiratory problems? What do you do, rub the patient's back?" But in fact, cardiopulmonary physiotherapy has been around for more than 100 years. The benefits of "movement and positioning" for health were first described in 1894 and a few years later, physicians realized that areas of atelectatic lung could be re-expanded with appropriate positioning and later still, in 1901, that gravity could be employed to assist the drainage of secretions from infected tuberculosis cavities. Since that time, the specialty of cardiopulmonary physiotherapy has continued to evolve and extend its boundaries to include the management of patients presenting with any medical problem including specific respiratory, cardiac and vascular disease, patients undergoing surgical intervention and those who are critically ill.

Cardiopulmonary physiotherapy is one of the core specialties of the profession; however, it is the only clinical area in which qualified physiotherapists often continue to practice, through participation with on-call rotas, long after specializing in another clinical area. As such, a sound theoretical and clinical foundation is essential.

Historically, students were taught cardiopulmonary physiotherapy using the "recipe" approach to treatment: this is how you treat a patient with asthma, this is how you treat a patient post myocardial infarction, this is how you treat a ventilated patient, and so on. However, thankfully this is no longer the case! Today, a problem-based approach is used, in which students are taught to undertake a thorough analytic assessment to identify physiological dysfunction, highlighting which problems may be amenable to physiotherapy. Clinical reasoning is then employed to identify a suitable treatment technique. There is no role for routine cardiopulmonary physiotherapy, so any intervention must be made following the prioritorized consideration of any concurrent problems and the patient's overall stability. Of course, the ability to do this successfully is totally dependent on the student having a sound grasp of both normal physiology and pathophysiology and dysfunction.

Learning the theory

As with any clinical specialty, it is absolutely essential for students to have a thorough understanding of normal structure and function, before being able to identify and consider the abnormal or pathologic. You wouldn't go to an outpatient setting to assess a patient with acute knee pain without knowing the structural anatomy of the knee joint and the interaction of the muscles acting over it. How can you decide which treatment technique is appropriate if you are unable to identify where and at what level dysfunction has occurred? In the same way, it is essential to have a good understanding of the structural anatomy of the thorax, heart, lungs and vasculature.

Physiotherapy students tend to fall into one of two camps: those who enjoy learning anatomy and find it easy to remember and those who prefer learning and understanding physiology. But like most aspects of the human body, the anatomy of the thorax, heart, lungs and vasculature is intrinsically linked to its physiology or function. Simplistically, anatomy is generally learning a fact, e.g. the heart has four chambers, whereas physiology requires a level of applied understanding, e.g. the four chambers of the heart contract and relax in a co-ordinated manner in order to move deoxygenated blood from the body through the lungs for oxygenation and carbon dioxide removal, ready to re-enter the systemic circulation. So you could say that anatomy provides the structural basis on which to understand physiology and therefore must be learnt first.

Tips for learning anatomy

Unfortunately, unlike the skeleton you got in order to learn musculoskeletal anatomy, you won't be given a heart and a set of lungs to keep in a box under your bed! Shame, because the visual memory of actually being able to handle something is a great aid to learning. It's much easier to remember the structure of an organ and how individual components interact when you can physically take it apart and reassemble it. This is particularly true of the heart and lungs, as most imaging of these organs provides a two-dimensional representation of what are three-dimensional structures. You may be at a university which offers you the chance to watch human cadaver dissection, which is a memorable event, to say the least; mainly as the smell of formaldehyde stays on your clothes for several hours after you leave, no matter how many times you wash your hands or spray your uniform with Febreze!® Alternatively, students have found exhibitions such as "Bodyworks®" useful for visualizing human anatomy. Virtual or three-dimensional interactive images are often available on the internet (e.g. www.anatomy.tv) but often require a license or subscription, which make them expensive for an individual but they may be available on campus. However, most universities have access to models of the heart and lungs which can be taken apart to reveal both external and internal structure.

Try drawing and labeling the anatomic structure of the heart, lungs, thorax and vasculature to reinforce learning and utilize visual memory. It is also a great way to self-test your understanding and recall. Use a skeleton to help understand how the typical and atypical ribs are different, and how that relates to their function. Look at the shape of the thorax and relate its structure to the normal mechanics of respiration.

When you start clinical placements, take every opportunity to watch any surgical procedure or clinical intervention. Cardiothoracic surgery is fabulous if you can watch, especially if you are able to stand at the "head end" and peer into the chest cavity. This is a wonderful way to visualize and consolidate anatomy; there is actually very little blood and it really helps to put structures into context. Don't touch anything covered in green surgical cloth or you will incur the wrath of the surgeon and his team, and if you feel faint or sick, always move away from the operating table as quickly as you can! Other clinical interventions such as bronchoscopy are also invaluable; being able to actually see inside the bronchial tree really helps to reinforce the structural anatomy of the airway and mucosa plus how these structures relate to function.

There is a wide range of "normal" in the general population, so the more "chests" you can review, the more familiar you will become with normal variation. Practice surface marking the heart and lungs on as many different people as you can and make sure you recruit both male and female models to practice on so you learn to accommodate for additional soft tissue! One good landmark to remember is in most cases the bra cup follows the line of the sixth rib.

Tips for learning physiology

Before embarking on learning physiology, remember to familiarize yourself with the anatomy first, as the structure of the cardiopulmonary system directly relates to its function. Remembering physiology is all about understanding; it is often sequential and may tell a story. Once you understand the story, remembering it becomes easier.

Writing your own flow diagrams of the key principles and points is a great way to condense the core information and also provides a fabulous revision tool for later on. This also works really well for learning pathology. Alternatively, read through each physiology lecture and pick out the top 10 points and bullet them in order. Learn the bullet points, which then act as a memory prompt to aid recall of the additional information.

The internet is an invaluable resource for learning normal physiology, pathology and dysfunction. Websites provide a wealth of simplistic explanations which have been written for the lay person. If there is an area you have difficulty in understanding, start by reading literature at this level. Once you have learnt the basics, increase the depth of your knowledge by using a more informative website aimed at undergraduate nurses or other allied health professionals. As your understanding grows, utilize literature and texts at a higher level, increasing the depth of your knowledge and understanding. Most physiology texts come with an accompanying CD which often provides a more visual approach to learning.

Tips for learning physiotherapy

All effective physiotherapy intervention aims to affect or reverse underlying physiological dysfunction. Therefore, in order to be able to use clinical reasoning to select an appropriate treatment, a thorough understanding of normal and abnormal physiology is required. You can't get away from the fact that you *have to know* the anatomy and physiology! Once you understand how an intervention, technique or adjunct works, then it can be "matched" to the physiological dysfunction identified on assessment. One textbook which students find very useful (Cardiopulmonary physiotherapy, Jones & Moffatt 2002) is written in this format; firstly common physiological dysfunction is identified and described, then possible intervention modalities which may be used in treatment are outlined with their key physiologic principles, supported by an evidence base.

Many universities have access to mannequins which can be used to practice manual hyperinflation and endotracheal suction, nasopharyngeal and oral suction and other physiotherapy intervention. Where available, use these resources to practice technique, because often the hardest aspect of something like endotracheal suction is actually getting a glove onto a nervous sweating hand, while holding the catheter under one arm and maintaining "aseptic or clean" technique, all under the scrutiny of the clinical educator!

Interactive DVDs, web-based sites and other media packages are very useful tools for learning physiotherapy techniques and skills; many DVDs and interactive CD-ROMs are available for loan from the BMA library or other similar outlets. Medical equipment manufacturers often produce fabulous interactive "teaching" packages to accompany their products. Try using a search engine to find an interactive site which may help you. Littmann® provides a comprehensive guide to auscultation and breath sounds (http://solutions.3m.com/wps/portal/ 3M/en_US/Littmann/stethoscope/education/educational-cd/lung-sounds/); similarly Dräger Medical® offers several excellent interactive teaching packages and down loads covering use of their mechanical ventilators (www.draeger.co.uk/MTms/internet/site/MS/internet/UK/ms/lib/Demos/int_lib_demo_evita.jsp).

BENCH TO BEDSIDE

Cardiopulmonary physiotherapy is an area where students often find it difficult to relate theory to practical application. It's hard to visualize the problems of a breathless patient if you have never seen one, never mind understanding how changing the patient's position may be of benefit. But most students report that as soon as they have used this knowledge on clinical placement, it all fits into place.

Preparation for clinical placement

This is where it gets really interesting! Analyzing the assessment of a cardiopulmonary patient is like doing a jigsaw, putting all the different pieces together to produce a clinical picture. Try to visualize the patient as a whole, thinking about how the body systems interact, rather than just thinking about the heart or lungs in isolation. Currently, cardiopulmonary physiotherapy is much more rehabilitation focused compared to the "shake 'n vac" image of old! Although physiotherapists tend to choose an area of clinical specialty, one of the skills of being an effective clinician is being able to think outside a diagnostic label and treat all presenting problems, whichever body system they may affect. All therapeutic intervention and clinical skills are transferable and can be applied as indicated.

For some students, undertaking a cardiopulmonary placement is the first time they have been faced with treating patients who are actually systemically ill or even dying. Often the patients are young or of a similar age to the student, which may add to any potential distress. Make sure you are able to develop a coping strategy, either using senior support, counseling or talking through difficult situations with friends. Remember that even though you may not be able to "cure" a patient, your intervention may improve their quality of life.

Cardiopulmonary placements can cover a vast range of clinical areas: general or specialist intensive care, medical or surgical high-dependency unit, medical wards, surgical wards, respiratory outpatients and community. For most students, a placement on the intensive care unit is particularly daunting, but actually it's one of the safest departments in the hospital; the patients are constantly monitored, receive one-to-one nursing and are surrounded by highly trained staff. It is also very unlikely you would be asked to treat a patient in this environment without supervision. Irrespective of which clinical setting you are working in, some core knowledge and skills are central and apply to all areas.

Always carry a notebook which can fit into your tunic pocket; it is invaluable for key information you may want to bring to or take away from the placement on a daily basis. Whichever level of training you are at, clinical educators will expect you to arrive on placement knowing how to undertake a cardiopulmonary assessment. Jot down the main points to include under "subjective" and "objective" headings in your notebook to act as a prompt if you feel nervous on the first day. Educators would prefer you used your initiative and were equipped with self-prompts, rather than staring at the floor or looking confused when unsure what to do! Always start by introducing yourself to the patient, explaining your role and what you would like to achieve. Go for the obvious first by gaining a subjective assessment of the patient. Develop an enigmatic smile to adopt when you ask your surgical patient "How are you?" and they reply with a 5-minute monologue of the change in their bowel habits! Look for the obvious signs of systemic illness: pyrexia, increased respiratory rate or an abnormal breathing pattern. It's much easier to remember these key points when you have a patient in front of you compared to "assessing" one of your symptom-free classmates in a tutorial. Try and develop your own "running order" for the assessment, then jot down the prompts in the corner of your notes so you can work through them steadily.

As part of the assessment procedure you should be able to auscultate (make sure the earpieces of the stethoscope are pointing forward or you won't hear anything at all!), get basic information from a chest X-ray and simple investigative tests. A list of commonly used drugs and their action is also a useful entry in your notebook.

Patients with cardiopulmonary problems present with one or more of five clinical problems, which are often intrinsically interlinked.

- Breathlessness
- Sputum retention
- V/Q mismatch
- Reduced lung volumes
- Deconditioning

The basic management of each one includes the use of appropriate positioning or exercise and some format of the active cycle of breathing techniques. Therefore, a good working knowledge of these interventions and how their application can be manipulated to treat these common problems is essential.

STETHOSCOPE

Once you start undertaking cardiopulmonary placements it's a good idea to buy your own stethoscope. There are many versions on the market which need careful consideration. For chest auscultation, the stethoscope must have several features: firstly, it must have a proper bell (flat stethoscopes are only suitable for taking blood pressures) which can be used to listen to different pitches of noise. The bell should feel heavy, so it can be placed securely on the patient's chest to limit extraneous noise and artefact. It's hard enough to accurately evaluate the noises you are meant to hear without the additional rustling of a lightweight bell again the patient's skin. The tubes must not be too long, so you can actually hear what is going on in the chest, but not so short that you end up with your nose under the patient's armpit when auscultating their chest. This is particularly important in intensive care when the ventilator and surrounding equipment produce so much noise (CXR may be more useful here); plus patients who have been unwell and nil by mouth for a prolonged period also have notoriously bad breath!

The Littmann® Classic II is a great starting point and can be purchased through many outlets and online sites including Amazon and e-Bay. Slightly cheaper stethoscopes are available but need to be thoroughly researched before purchase. Medscope offer a good alternative (www.medscope.co.uk/ acatalog/Doctors_Stethoscopes.html?gclid=CNKlsoOdhpYCFQyvQwodsObF Fg). If you are able to try a few out then do, as you may find the earpieces more comfortable in certain brands. Try and choose one in a vivid color – you will be able to spot it much more easily on the wards if you put it down. But most importantly, get your name engraved on the bell as soon as you have it: stethoscopes walk!

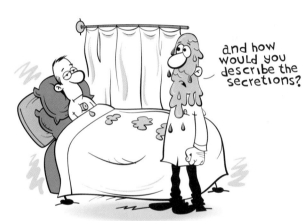

Tips for clinical placement

- Always have a spare uniform with you – this is the area where you are most likely to experience every bodily fluid known to man erupting with projectile precision at your tunic. Now you know why the trousers are so flared, so you can get them off quickly!

- Always wash your hands before and after handling a patient. Always adhere to any local infection control policy regarding apron, gloves, glasses, etc.

- Keep jewelery and anything pinned on your uniform to a minimum; you may scratch the patient or find yourself inadvertently attached to their hair when you move them, especially with babies and young children.

- Remove your watch before handling a patient.

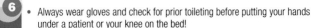

- Always wear gloves and check for prior toileting before putting your hands under a patient or your knee on the bed!
- Always adopt a holistic interprofessional approach to management which includes the patient and their families.
- Remember to explain every aspect of your treatment and how it may benefit the patient in order to gain "informed" consent.
- Get into the habit of talking to and including the patient in the treatment process, even if you don't think they can hear you.
- Always carry a notebook in your tunic pocket to write down anything you don't understand or are unfamiliar with, to look up later.
  - Names of conditions, drugs, procedures
  - References or titles of textbooks
  - Messages/liaison
  - How to bleep someone
  - Clinical educator's bleep number
  - Numbers and names of wards you are working on
  - Crash call number/fire alarm number for the hospital

Write key points in your notebook.

- Key points to remember for assessment
  - Subjective
  - Objective
  - Test results
- Components of ACBT
  - Breathing control
  - Lower thoracic expansion exercises ± manual techniques
  - Forced expiration technique
- CXR analysis
  - Technical assessment
  - Clinical assessment
  - Evaluation of film
- Auscultation
  - Earpieces must point forward to hear anything
  - When appropriate, always expose the thorax
  - Compare left to right
  - Listen through full respiratory cycle
  - Normal breath sounds
  - Added breath sounds and what causes them
  - Reduced breath sounds and what causes them
- Analysis of simple spirometry
  - FEV_1
  - FVC
  - FEV_1/FVC ratio

- PEFR
- Obstructive versus restrictive lung disease
- Ventilator modes
- Key points for indications and use of IPPB and CPAP
- Respiratory disease pathology
- Formulate your own glossary of terms

Laminate a small card containing the normal values you need to refer to on a regular basis.

- ABGs
- Cardiopulmonary values: HR, BP, CO, CI, CVP, PAOP, PAP, etc.
- Full blood count
- Electrolytes
- Urea and creatinine
- Always look at test results in series to view the trend of change
  - ABGs
  - CXR
  - Spirometry
  - Bloods
- Don't forget to use your hands! They are a valuable assessment tool.
- Don't be frightened to say you don't know or understand something; a proactive learner is preferable to one trying to wing it – ignorance may put a patient at risk.
- Foster a team approach, particularly in intensive care where other members of the team are experienced, skilled and knowledgeable.
- Be persuasive and explain the benefits of physiotherapy. Patients love to tell you "I've had major surgery, dear! I couldn't possibly get out of bed!"
- Always consider adequate analgesia. If the patient has pain, then your treatment cannot be fully effective.
- Get to know the ward clerk and administration staff. Knowing them is such an advantage when you need help finding staff, patients, telephone numbers, notes, test results and X-rays. Plus, more often than not, the chocolates are on their desk!!
- Always leave the bed space as you found it; good housekeeping is the best way to maintain good interprofession working!

Hazards of clinical placement

It's every student's nightmare: you start to mobilize a patient and only realize as they move away from the bed space that they are still attached to an arterial line transducer, which promptly self-destructs and emits a flow of blood comparable to Niagara Falls! There is blood all over you and the patient, and as you sheepishly ask for help, the junior doctor informs you with a steely glare that it took him 10 attempts to site the line in the first place.

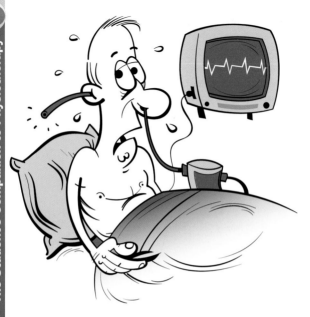

It sounds really obvious, but one of the most important things to consider before moving a patient is preparation of the bed space and surrounding area. Depending on the patient's presenting problems, they may be attached to no more than an oxygen mask and a saturation monitor or could have multiple lines, intercostal drains, wound drains, an epidural, a hemodialysis catheter and a patient-controlled analgesia pump. Although a rule of thumb suggests that the more lines and attachments in situ, the sicker the patient, as long as the patient is neurologically and hemodynamically stable they can still be moved and even mobilized. Even patients who are intubated and mechanically ventilated, but awake and stable, are still able to walk around the bed space within the limits of their tubing.

Take a few minutes to assess the site and location of all invasive lines; identify which can be transiently disconnected to facilitate mobility. Consider other external attachments such as ECG lines, oxygen masks and tubing, blood pressure cuff, oxygen saturation monitor. If the patient requires oxygen during mobilization, find a portable cylinder and attach the tubing. Remember to check that there is sufficient oxygen for the duration of your treatment. If the patient has intercostal drains in situ, think about whether they can be disconnected from external suction. Remember not to hold the drainage bottle above the site of insertion, otherwise the contents of the bottle will siphon back into the patient's chest! Once you are happy with the patient's state, prepare the immediate area. Patients who have been immobile will have reduced muscle strength and balance, increasing their likelihood of falling.

Don't be frightened to move the bed and other furniture to maximize space, especially if you and the patient are going to walk side by side. If you are in a side room and heading out to the main ward, open the door before starting to mobilize, as you may need to support the patient or carry a piece of equipment during mobilization. Consider carrying an oxygen saturation monitor if you are unsure how the patient will respond to exercise. Always ask for help if you are unsure or moving a patient for the first time.

EMERGENCY SITUATIONS

- If you do find yourself in the mist of a hemorrhaging artery, apply firm pressure to the area immediately and call for help.
  - Monitor vital signs.
- If you pull out an intercostal drain, block the insertion site with your hand. Apply pressure and call for help. If the patient is conscious, ask them to hold their breath or exhale until you occlude the hole to limit pneumothorax.
  - Monitor vital signs.
  - Auscultate chest.
- If you partially dislodge a line, notify the nursing or medical staff immediately and prevent any further traction on the line.
- If the patient inadvertently self-extubates, call for help immediately then assist ventilation with a resuscitation or Ambu-bag attached to a facemask until help arrives.
  - Monitor vital signs.
- Notify nursing or medical staff immediately if an endotracheal or tracheostomy tube becomes dislodged during treatment.
  - Monitor vital signs.

Student wisdom

"Know who is who! While on a critical care ward I was asked to help manually ventilate a patient while the ventilator pipes were untangled. I did so only to be interrupted by my clinical educator who informed me that the person I was helping was a student nurse ... she didn't know that I was a student physiotherapist: talk about the blind leading the blind! Critical care wards are not the place for shyness – if someone talks to you and you don't know who they are, ASK!" (Anon, Australia)

Conclusion

Cardiopulmonary physiotherapy is a fascinating, challenging and dynamic area in which to work. So if you were previously unaware that physiotherapists worked in intensive care or with patients who have cardiopulmonary disease, and the thought of sputum, blood and gore fills you with dread, try to keep an open mind until you have completed a couple of clinical placements. Many students are surprised just how much they enjoy this clinical specialty!

References

Jones, M., Moffatt, F., 2002. Cardiopulmonary Physiotherapy. Taylor and Francis, London.

Further reading

Bersten, A.D., Soni, N., Oh, T.E., 2003. Oh's Intensive Care Manual, fifth ed. Butterworth-Heinemann, London.

Foxall, F., 2008. Arterial Blood Gas Analysis: An Easy Learning System. M&K Publishing, Cumbria, UK.

Marieb, E.N., Hoehn, K., 2007. Human Anatomy and Physiology, seventh ed. Pearson, London.

Pryor, J., Prasad, A., 2008. Physiotherapy for Respiratory and Cardiac Conditions: Adults and Paediatrics (Physiotherapy Essentials), fourth ed. Churchill Livingstone, London.

Rowlands, A., Sargent, A., 2008. The ECG Workbook. M&K Publishing, Cumbria, UK.

West, J.B., 2007. Pulmonary Physiology and Pathophysiology, second ed. Lippincott, Williams and Wilkins, London.

West, J.B., 2008. Respiratory Physiology: The Essentials, eighth ed. Lippincott, Williams and Wilkins, London.

Neurologic physiotherapy
Nick Southorn

- Basics 83
- Conditions 85
- Assessment 86
- Treatment of the neurologic patient 88
- In the clinic 90

Studying physiotherapy

The first thing to say about neurologic physiotherapy is: don't panic! It may look daunting at first but once you learn the basics, the rest all falls into place. Having said that, neurology extends way beyond knowing the anatomy of the nervous system. Eventually (in the distant future), you will need intricate knowledge of association areas of the brain, the nervous system's response to damage – traumatic, pharmacologic, psychologic or pathologic – the role of the autonomic nervous systems, etc.

Additional reading for neurologic physiotherapy comes in the form of *Physical management in neurological rehabilitation* by Maria Stokes (2004). This is a particularly well-structured book that guides you through your learning in a very accessible way. Also available is *Neurological physiotherapy: a problem solving approach* by Susan Edwards (2002). This is a very nice book that is more concise with its fact delivery. It is exactly what it claims to be, though – a problem-solving book.

Neuro: more than most people think

Neurology is not just stroke rehabilitation – it encompasses anything with a neurologic element (which is most things). This is why, even if you never want to see a stroke patient, neurologic physiotherapy is a core area and one that must be understood.

This knowledge is vital if you are to understand your patient's condition, their prognosis, their goals, their potential and their experiences. Your knowledge will also link in with how you are affecting the nervous system. Are you getting the desired effect? Are you eliciting another effect that is not desirable (a side effect)? What is the mechanism and how do you work around it? If you are lucky enough to have a placement with neurologic physiotherapists, you will gaze in wonderment at their apparent ability to instinctively create a desirable action from the patient and how they utilize this movement. Please don't feel threatened by this: they are highly experienced clinicians and a great deal of their knowledge has evolved *after* qualification. It is a complex area and one that takes time to get the hang of.

What you need to know

Before you learn how physios treat neurologic conditions you need to acquire some basics.

- Brain anatomy and association areas
- The cranial nerves and function
- Ascending and descending spinal tracts and function
- The autonomic nervous system (parasympathetic, sympathetic and enteric)
- Dermatomes and myotomes (as in spinal levels of innervation)

Then start learning about the conditions that may present to a neurologic physiotherapist. As is the running theme in this book, these are the basic "must know" lists and will get you well grounded with knowledge.

- Stroke (cerebral vascular accident, CVA) – look at the different types and predisposing factors
- Traumatic brain injury (TBI)

- Motor neurone disease (MND)
- Peripheral nerve injuries
- Multiple sclerosis (MS)
- Parkinson's disease (PD)
- Huntington's disease
- Cerebral palsy (CP)
- Spina bifida

Then comes the treatment types. You will be expected to know about different treatment options available to patients regarding medical and surgical interventions as well as your more specialist knowledge of physiotherapeutic treatment. Treatment types include:

- vestibular and balance
- pain management
- exercise rehabilitation
- functional rehabilitation
- proprioceptive neuromuscular facilitation (PNF)
- orthotics and strapping.

Basics

Brain association areas are very important to get to grips with. As part of the diagnostic work-up, you will have a report detailing the area of a lesion of the brain. Neurologic physiotherapists know instinctively what the implications of that location are. An understanding of what the brainstem has to offer in comparison to the cerebellum and cerebrum will also help you relate injury to symptoms.

Learning about the brain usually results in a headache as you come across words that you know you will never remember the meaning of. However, if you take a methodologic approach (that's right, get the basics first) you will slowly get to grips with it all. The best bit of advice I had from a lecturer was: learning about the nervous system takes time. An example of progressive learning for the central nervous system is as follows.

The brain lies in the skull and is a mass of nerve bodies and axons. It is encased in a series of layers (externally inwards): the dura mater, arachnoid mater (encasing the subarachnoid space where large vessels lie), pia mater, gray matter and finally the white matter. Note the differences in the words "mater" and "matter." *Mater*, in this context, is apparently translated to mean "mother of the brain" (think of a mother cuddling her child) and *matter* is obviously as in "substance." The brain has two distinct sections – the cerebrum (the two large hemispheres at the top) and the cerebellum (the smaller bit posterior to the brainstem and inferior to the cerebrum).

The cerebral cortex has four lobes:

- frontal lobe (at the front)
- temporal lobe (think temple on the side of your head)
- occipital lobe (at the back)
- parietal lobe (at the back above the occipital lobe).

Pick one part at a time. For example, the frontal lobe plans sequences of response and controls emotions; it also has motor control over the eye muscles and speech. Look up Broca's area.

By having just that bit of information, you can already see that damage to the area may result in difficulty controlling emotions and communicating, while behavior deemed to be socially inappropriate may be displayed due to lack of discretion. This can be crudely described as losing the filter between the brain and the mouth as one may find someone lacking executive prowess (i.e. someone with frontal lobe damage) to be offensive.

So the point is that you work through the brain systematically, ensuring that you hit the right bits relevant to physiotherapy, such as:

- medulla
- corpus callosum
- pons
- midbrain
- basal ganglia connections (cortex, thalamus, globus pallidus, substantia nigra, caudate and putamen)
- blood supply – very important that you understand the circle of Willis.

Once you have the "brain" you can move on down the body and this includes the cranial nerves. You will remember their names due to the clever mnemonic discussed in Chapter 3. But what do they do? Fortunately, you will only have to develop a basic knowledge of these to begin with and build upon it if need be. The great thing about these is the fact that their names give away what they do (mostly anyway). To save you having to look these up, here they are.

I	Olfactory	Sense of smell
II	Optic	Visual information
III	Oculomotor	Eye movements
IV	Trochlear	More eye movements
V	Trigeminal	Sensations from the face and innervates mastication
VI	Abducens	Yet more eye movement
VII	Facial	Facial motor control, taste sensation and saliva production
VIII	Vestibulocochlear	Sound, rotation and gravity
IX	Glossopharyngeal	Taste sensation
X	Vagus	Most laryngeal and pharyngeal motor control
XI	Accessory	Neck muscles and shared function with the vagus
XII	Hypoglossal	Tongue muscles

Moving down the spinal column, we encounter a series of tracts. You should be able to identify the ascending and descending tracts and have a basic understanding of what information they carry (temperature, touch, pain, etc.). This is important for patients who have suffered a spinal trauma/incident whereby part of or all of the cord is disrupted.

The autonomic nervous system is made up of three parts and is called autonomic because it deals generally with the things that you do without conscious thought.

- Parasympathetic – rest and digest, the nonstressful situations
- Sympathetic – fight or flight, for when things get hairy
- Enteric – gut function (peristalsis) and gastric secretions

When you get into it, you may feel overwhelmed by it all. Many students liken neurology to learning a new language so it stands to reason that if you and your friends have many conversations about the anatomy and function of the central nervous system, you will eventually become fluent in it. Give it a go, you might be quite surprised!

Conditions

Learning about the conditions by now should be second nature. You get a condition, let's say multiple sclerosis, and you find the following.

ETIOLOGY (CAUSE)

An inflammatory autoimmune disorder of the CNS causing demyelinization of neurones, thus affecting the conductivity of these nerves.

EPIDEMIOLOGY

Temperate climates (i.e. not extremely cold or hot) exhibit higher incidences. More females to males are affected and the age range is 16–50.

PATHOLOGY

A nonself antigen replicates a protein in myelin, causing an autoimmune response, and the normal inflammatory pathways of adhesion molecules found in blood vessel endothelium allow transportation to the CNS where the myelin sheath is degenerated. The perpetuation is a result of oligodendrocyte death which, in turn, affects other myelin sheaths corresponding to other axons. The resulting absence of salutatory conduction slows the conduction of action potentials to the extent that they effectively cease.

CLINICAL (PRESENTING) FEATURES

- Symptoms arise and resolve periodically
- Frequent urination/incontinence
- Ataxia
- Weakness in lower limbs (spastic weakness)
- Impotence
- Unilateral eye dysfunction – demyelination of the optic nerve (CN II)

DIFFERENTIAL DIAGNOSIS

These can usually be excluded by questioning and a good history.

- Vitamin B12 deficit (can cause visual loss and spastic weakness along with peripheral neuropathy)
- Spinal cord compression (causes lower limb weakness and urinary disorders such as urinary retention)
- Space-occupying lesion in the brain or spinal cord
- Hereditary spastic weakness
- HIV

TREATMENT

- Some immune modulators are effective at decreasing the frequency of episodes.
- The mainstay of treatment is managing symptoms, such as using baclofen for spasticity, laxatives for constipation, antidepressants and psychotherapy for low mood, analgesia for pain, etc.
- Physiotherapy is also a symptomatic treatment for movement and functional loss. Other options open to the physio are pain management and spasticity control to minimize abnormal tone, prevent contractures and encourage weight bearing and independence. As with all treatments, an educational/motivational role is also key as the patient must be aware of the disease progression in order to remain realistic regarding targets, etc.

So that is a basic knowledge base on MS. I would now create a knowledge tree and highlight any term that I am not 100% clear on and look it up. In the natural progress of your learning, you may want to add other headings that capture your imagination, like "drugs," "contraindications to therapy," "three most recent research papers relating to treatment," etc.

Assessment

The assessment of the neurologic patient will depend on the condition you are about to see. Largely, you will be expected to extract the usual assessment information such as past medical history, history of present complaint, social history, etc. But you already know that by now!

Things that you may want to learn about in assessments in general include the following.

DERMATOMES

- Sensation – is it normal or hyperesthetic? Is there altered sensation such as burning or pins and needles?
- Heat/cold – again, is it a normal reaction to temperature?
- Touch discrimination – can the patient discriminate between two points at varying distances apart?

MYOTOMES

- Strength of contraction (see Chapter 10 for strength measures)
- Reflexes – are they rather too brisk? Do they exist at all?

MUSCLE BULK

- Are the muscles atrophied/hypertrophied?

SWELLING/EDEMA

- Are the ankles swollen? Why would this be?

PROPRIOCEPTION/BALANCE

- Is it intact? How can you tell?
- Remember that upper limb proprioception may be tested too!
- See the BERG Balance Scale in Chapter 10.

CO-ORDINATION

- Finger-to-nose test
- Heel-to-shin test

GAIT

OTHER FUNCTIONS

- Hand to mouth (feeding)
- Hand to head (combing hair, scratching head)
- Hand behind back (unclasping a bra)
- Putting on footwear

In terms of measuring joint ranges for all joints, something that is time consuming and generally not a great experience for the patient, some practitioners prefer to stick to the functional objectives mentioned above. This is especially true in stroke rehabilitation where the patient may not be interested in hearing that he has gained an extra 5° elbow flexion but rather more engaged with hearing that he is much closer to being able to feed himself again. The message here is: make the objective markers relevant to the patient!

Treatment of the neurologic patient

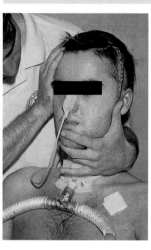

Fig. 7.1 Some neurological patients will have much higher needs than others. With kind permission from Elsevier. This photo was published in Edwards S (2002) *Neurological Physiotherapy* (2nd Ed) Edinburgh: Churchill Livingstone (p. 6.14).

How to manually handle neurologic patients is one of the physiotherapist's key areas of knowledge. All those joints you now know about that are supported by muscles may be completely vulnerable due to lack of tone in those supporting muscles. Speaking of tone – if you go at a neurocompromised patient in the wrong way you will send their tone through the roof and any further attempts at physiotherapy treatment will be pointless for a while. On the other hand, purposefully increasing tone in a controlled way can be therapeutic. See, it is complicated.

Pediatrics is a special area of neurology and a reasonable understanding of the pathophysiologic processes involved in the childhood syndromes and diseases is necessary. See Chapter 10 for more information.

Specific treatments should be noted. You may be expected to attend your clinical placement with an understanding of the treatment types. The following list is from Stokes (2004) and all should be researched further for more detail.

- Brushing – for facilitation of muscle contraction.
- Ice (short period of application) – for facilitation of motor response.
- Ice (long period of application) – reduction of afferent and efferent neurotransmission.
- Tapping – light tapping over a tendon to elicit a contraction.
- Fast passive stretch – again, to elicit a contraction via autogenic contraction (stretch reflex).
- Joint compression – stimulation of mechanoreceptors for enhanced proprioception.
- Vibration – high frequency (100–300 Hz), low amplitude for facilitation of sustained contraction, depression of the antagonistic muscle motoneurones and depression of the stretch reflex of the muscle.

- Vestibular stimulation – manipulation of the motor system by gross movement.
- Slow passive stretch – promotion of muscle relaxation via the Golgi apparatus.
- Splinting – posture maintenance/prolonged passive stretch.
- Positioning – specialist knowledge of positioning to reduce tone, contractures and discomfort.
- Hydrotherapy – exercise and movement in the supportive surroundings of water. The therapeutic effect of hydrotherapy is really worth getting to grips with.
- Gym ball – challenging the dynamic control of the patient is amongst the many uses of the gym ball.
- Proprioceptive neuromuscular facilitation (PNF) – use of diagonal patterns against manual resistance.
- Cardiovascular exercise and strength training – a controversial but ever more popular treatment for neurologic conditions due to the emerging supporting evidence.
- Electrical stimulation – use of electricity for pain relief (such as TENS) and management of spasticity. Electrical stimulation of muscle may also be used.

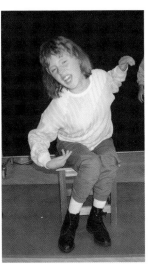

Fig. 7.2 Promoting independent balance plays a significant part of neurological physiotherapy" With kind permission from Elsevier. This photo was published in Edwards S (2002) *Neurological Physiotherapy* (2nd Ed) Edinburgh: Churchill Livingstone (p. 192)

"TOOL BOX"

- Tendon hammer
- Sharp/soft tool
- Warm/cool tool
- Point discrimination tool (a wheel with many points at varying distances) although these should be available in the hospital

In the clinic

One aspect that you need to remember in neurology all the time is manual handling. The rules are completely different with neuro patients. If you can turn up with an awareness of how to approach and handle patients with each condition, your clinical educator will adore you! Another aspect of this area is understanding the roles of your fellow professionals, as with most areas of physiotherapy. As a basic guide, here are just a few.

CHIROPODIST/PODIATRIST

Podiatrists work to improve the mobility, independence and the quality of life for their patients by providing preventive care, diagnosis and treatment of a wide range of problems affecting the feet, ankles and lower limb (Society of Chiropodists and Podiatrists 2009). With neurologic conditions, the integrity of the feet is invariably affected and thus a podiatrist is needed to ensure they are kept in immaculate condition and to treat any conditions that present, including immobility, weakness and joint laxity (where physiotherapy and podiatry may overlap a little).

MEDIC

A medical doctor oversees the medical aspects of care for the patient while being mindful of other potential issues for which to bring in another specialist.

NURSE

The nurse's role depends on who they are! Some nurses ensure the patients are comfortable, some that they receive the prescribed medication on time, some co-ordinate the patient's stay from admission to discharge (a hugely complex role that involves making everyone happy). Some nurses take on more of a clinician role in, say, mental heath or respiratory medicine. Whatever their role, the nurse typically spends more time with the patient than anyone else and therefore is a good person to ask for help.

OCCUPATIONAL THERAPY (OT)

Occupational therapists work with people who have physical, mental and/or social problems, either from birth or as a result of accident, illness or aging. Their aim is to enable people to achieve as much as they can for themselves, so they get the most out of life. When people cannot do things which are important to them – such as getting dressed, having a shower, going to work, socializing or undertaking a favorite hobby – an occupational therapist can help them in many ways, based on each individual person's needs and lifestyle (College of Occupational Therapy 2008).

PSYCHOLOGIST

Psychology is the scientific study of people, the mind and behavior. It is both a thriving academic discipline and a vital professional practice (British Psychological Society 2009). Psychologists employ a broad range of techniques tailored to each individual patient. In neurologic rehabilitation, they are immensely important to help the patient come to terms with whatever happened and move forward. Note: a *psychiatrist* is a medical doctor who specializes in psychologic issues and may prescribe medicines as treatment.

SPEECH AND LANGUAGE THERAPY/PATHOLOGY (SLT)

Speech and language therapists are allied health professionals. They work with children and adults who have difficulties with communication, or with eating, drinking and swallowing (Royal College of Speech and Language Therapists 2009).

In conclusion, you will need to acquire knowledge that will allow you to understand the patient's condition, assess the situation and develop a rehab prognosis. Only then can you begin to apply your treatment expertise in order to achieve the maximum possible potential for the patient.

> **Student wisdom**
>
> "Always have in mind that when learning from books about neurologic physiotherapy that you will never get the full picture until you meet neurologic patients. That is when it all falls into place and you really begin to cement your knowledge and handling skills together." (Anon, USA)

References

British Psychological Society, 2009. Homepage. Available at: <www.bps.org.uk>.

College of Occupational Therapy, 2008. About OT. Available at: <www.cot.co.uk/public/aboutus/intro/what.php>.

Edwards, S. (Ed.), 2002. Neurological Physiotherapy: A Problem Solving Approach, second ed. Churchill Livingstone, Edinburgh.

Royal College of Speech and Language Therapists, 2009. Homepage. Available at: <www.rcslt.org>.

Society of Chiropodists and Podiatrists, 2009. Homepage. Available at: <www.feetforlife.org>.

Stokes, M. (Ed.), 2004. Physical Management in Neurological Rehabilitation, second ed. Mosby, Edinburgh.

Pharmacology
Nick Southorn

- How do I get my head around all of this?   94
- It's all about class!   95
- What do I need to know about these drugs?   97
- In the clinic   98
- Conclusion   98

Studying physiotherapy

Pharmacology is the study of drugs and their interactions within the body. It is a very important area to get to grips with as you will be seeing these medications used on a regular basis. As it stands at the time of writing, few UK physio schools teach detailed pharmacology as UK physiotherapists don't have medical prescribing rights unless they undertake postgraduate training. In most other developed countries physios do study pharmacology, not to presume a career in prescribing medications but to prepare the physiotherapist with the skills needed to develop a clear clinical picture from knowing the medicines taken by the patient. Also, some drugs do contraindicate physiotherapy treatments. For example, long-term steroid use can lead to thin skin and low bone density; anticoagulation therapy can make a patient prone to bleeding, etc. Your lecturers will guide you about what is expected from you regarding this topic. It is a complex area to get to grips with but also fascinating once you get into it. You don't need any specialist tools as such except a vivid imagination to bring to life the intricate interactions of these chemicals.

How do I get my head around all of this?

Good question! You will already have an understanding of the normal physiologic workings of the human body and the pathologic processes of common conditions – inflammation, for example (and if it's all a bit vague, pharmacology is a good topic to remind you what physiology is all about). Understanding the drugs is literally working out how they reduce the symptoms of that pathology – they do it by either disease modification or symptom management. For this reason it is strongly advised that "pharmacology" is studied *within* study relating to disease. As a physio you will not be expected to be a font of all knowledge regarding medicine – that is why we have doctors! With that in mind, allow yourself to be satisfied with a general knowledge of the drugs rather than the complexities.

It is usually a good idea in any case to develop your own "glossary of words/ terms" for pharmacology to help you get to grips with it all. This may sound time consuming but just have a look at how simple the definitions can be in order to have a decent effect. Any glossary should only have a "reminder" rather than a full description.

- Opioid
  - Any substance that binds to an endogenous (within the body) opioid receptor antagonistically. They are both neurotransmitters and neurohormones producing both inhibition (expressed as analgesia in the spinal cord) and excitation (expressed as nausea in the chemoreceptor trigger zone). They may be *endogenous* (produced within the body) or *exogenous* (administered for the purpose of analgesia).
- Receptor agonist
  - A drug that binds to a receptor and stimulates it.
- Receptor antagonist
  - A drug that binds to a receptor site, preventing others from doing so. It typically has no effect itself other than as a barrier to the receptor site.

- Potency
  - The dose of a drug needed to produce the desired effect (Stannard & Booth 2004).

Learn about the advantages and disadvantages of administration such as:

- oral (pills, liquid, etc.)
- intravenous (IV)
- transdermal (patches)
- rectal (suppositories)
- inhaled
- subcutaneous
- buccal (under the top lip)
- epidural, subarachnoid.

There are two ways really of studying about medicine: learning about the *class* of drug, i.e. how the *types* of drug work and the names of the drugs that fall into that class; and learning about the *specific* drug and to what class it belongs. Either way, you will find it gets easier as you go along as more and more drugs belong to the same class.

It is difficult to explain the difference between the two. Learning about the class will ensure that the prominent detail of your learning is the science of the drug whereas learning the names and action will ensure you know what that drug does but perhaps fail to recall the later learned details of how it works. It is for that reason that I can say that if you have an interest in pharmacology and medical physiology, or if your course requires it, you will find learning about the biochemistry of medicine fascinating and worth while. However, if medication is not your interest (and perhaps that is the reason you became a physiotherapist and not a doctor) then learn the names and the basic action – that will suit you much better. The net result is essentially the same – you see you patient is taking simvastatin and you can confidently predict that he has high cholesterol!

It's all about class!

If you fancy giving the class system a go then the good news is that you only need to learn a few of them – the rest you can pick up as you go. Here is a list of the most popular types that you may wish to investigate further. Some people define the class of a drug by its effect – antihypertensive, antibiotic, bronchodilator – and some by its pharmacologic action: beta-blocker, ACE inhibitor (both antihypertensive medication), etc. For simplicity I will opt for the former: class by effect.

Here are just a few that you might want to get to grips with as you will be seeing them regularly.

ANALGESIC/ANTI-INFLAMMATORY

- NSAIDs
- Steroids
- Opioids
- Nonopoids

ANTICOAGULANT

ANTIMICROBIAL

- Antibiotics
- Antivirals
- Antifungals

ANTIDEPRESSANT

- Serotonin selective reuptake inhibitors (SSRIs)
- Tricyclics
- Monoamine oxidase inhibitors

ANTIDIABETIC

- Insulin
- Sulphonylureas
- Biguanides

ANTIHYPERTENSIVE

- Angiotensin-converting enzyme (ACE) inhibitors
- Beta-blockers
- Calcium channel blockers

BRONCHODILATOR

- Adrenoreceptor agonists
- Antimuscarinic (aka anticholinergic)

DIURETIC

- Thiazide
- Loop
- Potassium sparing
- Osmotic

THROMBOLYTICS

Of course, there are disease-specific drugs that you may want to research, such as those used in the treatment of Parkinson's disease (PD), as they don't fit a typical class so you might want to consider "anti-Parkinson's disease" drugs as a class! You will come across plenty that act upon certain systems and structures such as the parasympathetic nervous system, synapses, endocrine function, etc. and therefore a previous knowledge of these is important. What this also means is that the more you cover, the easier and more familiar it will all become.

What do I need to know about these drugs?

This is very dependent on what drugs you are likely to come across. For example, in the USA physiotherapists do not provide respiratory support in the same way physiotherapists do in Britain and thus if you take bronchodilators as an example, you'd be expected to know considerable pharmacologic detail in the UK, and perhaps the more practical aspects of the delivery of the drug, i.e. why, how, when, in the States.

Your tutors/clinical educators, etc. may guide you on this but you might consider pain management, cardiorespiratory medicine and neurologic management medicine to be core pharmacologic subjects of which to have a detailed knowledge.

So, for an example of how you might approach learning about a class of drug, I will use nonsteroidal anti-inflammatory drugs (NSAIDs), a class of drug that all physiotherapists should know about. Again, it is assumed that a physiologic knowledge exists, specifically that prostaglandin sensitizes the peripheral nerves to chemical and mechanical stress resulting in nociception and the sensation of pain, and that prostaglandin production depends upon the function of cyclo-oxygenase (COX) to metabolize arachidonic acid (Ganong 1995).

NSAIDS

Probably the most prescribed class of drugs in the world; it is estimated that 30 million people take an NSAID *each day!* (Stannard & Booth 2004). The action is largely attributed to COX inhibition; however, Stannard & Booth (2004) cite the interaction with endogenous opioid systems, inhibition of neutrophil activation, and an action at the spinal level reducing the effect of "wind up."

Most NSAIDs will reach their peak therapeutic range within 2 hours.

Drug names: ibuprofen, diclofenac, naproxen, etc.

Ibuprofen

- *What is it?* A propionic acid NSAID.

- *How is it available?* Without medical prescription in tablet form (syrup for children).

- *Normal dose.* 400 mg three times/day (1.2 g daily) for adults as an over-the-counter dose. However, can be prescribed at higher doses up to 2.4 g daily: 6×400 mg tablets (BMJ RPS 2007). Ibuprofen is usually taken after meals to reduce side effects.

- *How does it work?* COX inhibition. However, ibuprofen is not COX-2 specific so some side effects of COX-1 inhibition may be experienced such as increased gastric secretion.

- *Side effects.* Gastrointestinal discomfort including excessive acid secretion to the stomach. The *British National Formulary 54* (BMJ RPS 2007) also cites nausea, diarrhea, bronchospasm, headache, depression and insomnia. It is noteworthy that the majority of patients experience very few actual ill effects. If a patient of yours is suspected of having any of these side effects tell them to visit their family doctor.

* *Contraindications.* Heart failure, asthma, pregnancy and breast feeding. Use in the elderly is under caution.
* *Brand/other names.* You get the idea now …

Of course, you would then do the same for the other drugs identified above, each one becoming slightly easier as more similarities become apparent between them.

Other drugs that you may come across but may not need to know much about just require the basics, such as:

METOCLOPRAMIDE HYDROCHLORIDE

* *What is it?* Antiemetic (helps prevent feeling/being sick).
* *How is it available?* Prescription only.
* *How does it act?* Centrally and noncentrally (directly on the GI tract).
* *Indications.* Nausea/vomiting due to GI disorders, vertigo, and drug induced (opioid, chemotherapy).
* *Physio relevance.* None, i.e. this drug will have no impact on therapy.

See … simple!

All in all, pharmacology fits nicely into your knowledge of physiology. In many ways it really enhances your physiologic knowledge as you begin to explore the realms of biochemistry.

In the clinic

The great thing about learning about drugs is that you can always carry some form of aide mémoire to help you, from just a few notes in your pocket to the pocket guide (Kenyon & Kenyon 2009) to the *British National Formulary* (BNF) to the American Drug Index! If you are unsure as to what a drug is, don't panic, just asterisk it and look it up. NEVER try to bluff your way through a conversation and pretend you know more than you do as it will never end well.

You might find that a wise move is to make a list of the top 10 drugs used regularly in each area and make your own reminder sheet (e.g. musculo-skeletal: paracetamol, NSAIDs, hot/cold creams, etc; respiratory: broncho-dilators, inhaled steroids, antihypertensive, diuretics, etc.).

Conclusion

Pharmacology, drugs, medicine, etc. … it really is what you make of it. If your course demands a detailed knowledge then I hope this guide will help you develop your understanding. It is worth only going to the depth that is required for now to save yourself additional stress; you can always add to it later.

References

British Medical Journal (BMJ) and Royal Pharmaceutical Society (RPS), 2007. British National Formulary 54. British Medical Journal and Royal Pharmaceutical Society, London.

Ganong, W.F., 1995. Review of Medical Physiology. Appleton and Lange, Connecticut.

Kenyon, J., Kenyon, K., 2009. The Physiotherapist's Pocket Book: Essential Facts at Your Finger Tips, second ed. Churchill Livingstone, Edinburgh.

Stannard, C., Booth, S., 2004. Pain, second ed. Churchill Livingstone, Edinburgh.

Pharmacology

9

Biopsychosocial approach
Paul Watson

- Why a biopscyhosocial perspective?   102
- A biopsychosocial model of pain disability   103
- In the clinic   107
- Conclusion   109

Studying physiotherapy

John was 44. A year ago he developed low back pain following a particularly heavy day at work when he moved about 40 25 kg bags of cement off a lorry. His low back was painful the next day. Despite treatment his back pain got worse; he stopped work and started walking with elbow crutches. Routine physiotherapy did not help him. He presented in my clinic unable to walk more than 10 meters without his crutches and no more than 100 meters with them. His range of motion of the spine was severely limited and he was unable to lie flat on the plinth for assessment. His MRI scan demonstrated minor degenerative changes at L4–5 but nothing else; neurology was normal and all blood tests were normal.

Jim was also 44. He had repeated episodes of low back pain and leg pains over 10 years. A year ago he had a particularly bad episode and suffered loss of sensation and movement in his left foot. He had surgery and a diskectomy. Following surgery he developed a dropped foot and neuropathic pain in his lower leg. He returned to work as a kitchen fitter but 2 months ago experienced another episode of back pain while maneuvring a large cooker. He received extra analgesia from his GP but no advice on exercise or work so Jim started swimming and gentle cycling to help maintain his lumbar fitness. His last scan demonstrated degenerative changes throughout the lumbar spine with a large disk prolapse centrally at L2–3 and a small one on the right at L3–4. Jim's main reason for attending clinic was to get advice on returning to work.

Why a biopscyhosocial perspective?

John and Jim both have back pain as the main reason for consulting but their presentation could not be more different. Obviously the clinical assessment cannot explain the differences and imaging does not explain the severity of pain. It might be easy to simply classify Jim as stoical or motivated and John as weak or unmotivated but those pejorative terms are no use clinically and do not help explain *why* they are so different. For this we must look to explanations other than the biomedical model.

The foundations of a biomedical approach to disease were laid by Virchow in the early 19th century (Virchow 1858). In this model one first examines the body for signs of abnormal pathology, infers the cause of the disease from the observations, applies a treatment and expects the signs of disease to improve. This works well for isolated pathology but it was incorrectly extrapolated from signs of disease to the cause of disability. A biomedical model of disability is predicated on there being a linear relationship between the cause of the illness, the pathology identified, the severity of the symptoms, the degree of functional limitation and the consequent disability. The simple cure was to address the root cause and everything else would improve of its own accord. However, things are not that simple. In everyday life we know of people who seem to be very disabled by relatively moderate illnesses and complaints and those who despite pain and/or physical impairment do not let it interfere with their ability to work or conduct their hobbies. As you meet patients you will no doubt become aware that some seem to "keep going" despite considerable problems whereas other seem defeated by the same condition and become very disabled and dependent on the help of others.

So what is it that makes people with similar conditions and similar levels of disease so different in their physical function and disability? In the most simple of concepts, it is what people understand and believe about their condition, the way they cope with the condition and their own perception of their ability to be able to do things despite their illness/impairment. The relative contribution of examination (clinical testing, MRI), physical findings (muscle strength, range of motion) or even physiologic tests in nonpain conditions (blood gases, cardiorespiratory disease) varies by condition but in most, nonclinical, mainly psychologic and social factors are important or pre-eminent in explaining the level of disability (Main et al 2008).

Unfortunately, over-reliance on a biomedical model of pain results in patients being classified as malingering or exaggerating their symptoms for secondary gain such as access to benefits or to avoid work or unpleasant circumstances. This does our patients a disservice. And it is not just the medical profession who do this. The same may happen if physiotherapists have an overly biomedical or biomechanical model of musculoskeletal pain.

In order to manage people better we must address the biomedical/ biomechanical factors *and* the psychosocial.

A biopsychosocial model of pain disability

It is important to note that this chapter refers to pain-related disability and not to the perception or reporting of pain as a sensation. This in itself is an interesting subject but here I will concentrate on disability resulting from pain.

Some of the most complete research comes from the musculoskeletal field, particularly low back pain. In this area, not only are we able to look at the factors which are most important in determining the degree of disability but longitudinal studies have demonstrated that psychosocial factors can predict the likelihood of disability over a year after onset. One of the reasons why psychosocial influences in musculoskeletal pain are so well researched is that we cannot externally corroborate a person's pain, we only have their report to go on. The intensity of pain in chronic pain conditions has often been reported to explain relatively little about disability. Studies have demonstrated that pain explains, at best, about 24% of the disability of people attending physiotherapy for back pain (Woby et al 2007); in tertiary care centers like pain management programs, it might explain 8% or less of disability (Turner et al 2000).

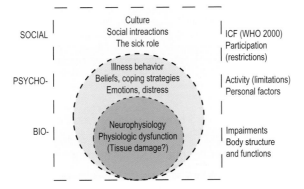

Fig. 9.1 The Glasgow Biopsychosocial model for low back pain. (Reproduced from Waddell 2004, with kind permission from Elsevier.)

A biopscyhosocial model for pain was developed by Waddell (2004) (see Fig. 9.1); at the core of the model is the perception of a sensation which is nociceptive or interpreted as potentially damaging. We then try to make sense of this sensation. Is it damaging? Do we need to be concerned? Our interpretation/cognitions about the sensation influence our emotional reaction to it; this is the affective component. This interpretation influences what we do about the pain – our pain or illness *behavior*. If we think it is nothing and it will go away by itself, we generally do little, are unconcerned and carry on. However, we might believe that it is a sign of damage and requires treatment and therefore will consult a healthcare practitioner. All our understanding of health and illness and our reactions to this are influenced by our prior experience, learning and influences from the social environment, e.g. what is acceptable and unacceptable illness behavior for a particular problem (Main et al 2008). Illness behavior is everything we do with regard to a condition, including reporting pain, taking medication, vocalizing, body posture and movement, adopting a sick role and seeking economic benefits (sick pay, social security benefits) (Keefe & Dunsmore 1992).

So what are the important things to consider?

Space prevents a detailed analysis of all the influences on pain-related disability and the interactions here. I recommend you read a good general textbook such as *The back pain revolution* by Waddell (2004) or *Pain management* by Main et al (2008). Here I will, of necessity, give just a broad review of the main features.

They can really be put into the following main areas but all of these interlink and overlap and cannot really be seen as completely distinct.

Hypervigilance to somatic sensations is a propensity to notice and focus on a symptom or body part which one is concerned about or which is painful where one perceives a threat (Crombez et al 1999). Our vigilance to sensory events is shaped by the importance (threat value) we give them; the more important we feel they are, the more likely they are to draw our attention. As such, hypervigilance is part of attentional processing.

Increased attention to sensations might be driven by threatening health information, that a particular pain is associated with injury or serious disease, for example. A person who injures their back and who finds certain movements painful is likely to be vigilant of the sensations in their back as they change posture; they may constantly monitor it for changes in sensation. The threat value of the sensation, i.e. an incorrect movement may cause pain, focuses their attention. This makes them more likely to interpret sensations as potentially damaging. Much of the work in this area has been conducted by Crombez and colleagues who demonstrated that chronic pain patients who were hypervigilant to pain not only had a lower threshold for detecting an experimental stimulus, they also had lower pain thresholds (see Van Damme et al 2004 and Crombez et al 2005 for reviews). Hypervigilant patients were also likely to be more disabled.

BELIEFS ABOUT THE CONDITION AND TREATMENTS

The component parts are difficult to separate out. Beliefs are pre-existing views of an illness or condition shaped by our previous experience, social and cultural history (Main et al 2008). If you believe that back pain is a sign of a serious condition which must be rested then you are more likely to rest as a way of managing it. If you believe that back pain requires a MRI scan, you are more likely to demand one and less likely to engage in physiotherapy unless you have had one. In short, beliefs drive behavior.

Expectancies are our beliefs about the future course of a condition – that it will progress or it will be time limited, it will result in increased disability or in only temporary restriction. Our interpretation will influence our behavior as we try and manage the expected future. Expectancies also color our perception of our own role in managing our condition. A patient might expect that it is the physiotherapist's job to fix them, for example, and not their own.

Outcome expectancies are the perception of the likely outcome of the condition irrespective of the patient's view of their own ability to influence the future. For example, a patient might have the impression that they have a progressive degenerative disease of the intervertebral disks which will need spinal fusion in the future. This rather bleak picture is unlikely to spur many people into exercise and self-management if they believe the outcome is inevitable and beyond their influence.

Self-efficacy is the belief that a person has the skill or ability to do something (behavior) in order to produce a desired outcome (Bandura 1977), and that the behavior will actually result in a desired outcome. For example, a person with back pain might believe that they are able to control their pain by regulating their activities (pacing) and that this will lead to increased activity without an increase in pain (Asghari & Nicholas 2001). Of course, the opposite can apply: a patient might think that he cannot exercise and exercise will not lead to an improvement; in fact, he might believe increased exercise might lead to a worsening of his condition.

People who are low in self-efficacy are less likely to acquire self-management skills or indeed may be less likely to see self-management, in the form of exercise or increasing physical activities, as a way of managing their condition. Much of our rehabilitation requires the patient to take on a self-management role. We cannot supervise their exercises day to day so we must instil in them the belief that they have the ability to help themselves and that to do so will lead to an improvement in their condition (Woby et al 2008).

SPECIFIC FEARS ABOUT HURT AND HARM

Most of the research in this area has been in musculoskeletal pain but pain-related behavior can be seen in other patients, for example after a myocardial infarction, and can be a powerful determinant of the patient's behavior. The fear/avoidance model of pain suggests that we avoid activities which we fear will be harmful and this avoidance in turn leads to increased disability as patients restrict their activities more and more (Vlaeyen & Linton 2000). In the case of low back pain, some people have actually suggested that fear of pain changes muscle recruitment and this in turn may leave the spine vulnerable to damage or increased nociception (Moseley & Hodges 2006).

Most people are simply wary of physical activity because in the past it has resulted in increased symptoms. However, there is a subgroup of patients who are so afraid of physical activity that they might be seen as having a phobic reaction to activity. This reaction is specific to certain types of activity. Vlaeyen et al (2002a) have suggested specifically identifying the types of activities that patients might be fearful of, which can be done using simple photographs (Leeuw et al 2007). Physiotherapists should always remember that patients' fears might seem irrational as they are influenced by the patient's own personal experience rather than the biomechanical demands of a particular task or the potential for harm as the physiotherapist sees it. The longer avoidance of activities persists, the more disabled a person is likely to become. There is now a large body of work demonstrating that fear-avoidant patients are more disabled and report more disability than those who are not. It may be one of the most important psychosocial factors maintaining disability in patients attending physiotherapy for low back pain, and reducing fear of activity seems to be very influential in the process of reducing disability through physiotherapy pain management approaches (Woby et al 2008).

Increased disability and avoidance of activity, especially valued activities such as work, hobbies and social activities with friends and family, increase the interference of the pain into the patient's life (Morley 2008). This can lead to reduced social interaction, loss of employment and eventual low mood and even depression which in itself can make the perception of disability greater. Many physiotherapists believe that managing depression or low mood is not in their domain of treatment but by enabling the patient to re-engage in valued activities, increase social interaction and return to work, we can help to improve mood. Consequentially this must form part of goal planning with the patient (Main et al 2008).

COPING STYLES AND STRATEGIES

Coping with pain is a dynamic process in which the patient tries to find the best way to cope with their pain and disability. It will of course be heavily influenced by all the factors above. Many years ago, Letham et al (1983) referred to patients as confronters and avoiders. Avoiders manage their pain by not engaging in any activity they think might be detrimental. The confronters carry on as usual, possibly by using exercise, activity regulation (pacing) and medication to help them. Sometimes this is effective but occasionally the business-as-usual approach can lead to overactivity with eventual failure. However, confronters might not just carry on regardless – they may realize the limitations caused by their problem and effectively adjust or accommodate to the problem by changing their goals and expectations. For example, a 45-year-old man might realize that his shoulder pain is being made worse by playing rugby so he stops this and takes up another less demanding sport which he finds equally enjoyable.

Coping strategies are the actions people take to deal with the situation and are sometimes classed as active and passive, although the concept of any coping strategy as passive is contested in the literature as no *action* can really be deemed *passive*. In more recent years, one of the most important negative coping strategies to receive attention is catastrophizing, which is a negative bias in processing information (Sullivan et al 2001). This is a cognitive distortion which leads the individual to attend to negative or threatening information and/or to process events negatively. A patient who catastrophizes is more likely to believe that they have a serious condition and that the outcome will be bleak, e.g. that they will never be able to work again, that they will require a wheelchair in the future. There is an unintentional selective attention to information which reinforces these beliefs at the expense of more positive information and evidence. Such patients are also more likely to see an increase in their pain as a sign of a worsening condition.

Positive coping strategies include diverting attention (keeping busy so as not to notice the pain) and increasing activity. Other negative strategies include avoiding activity and passively hoping the pain will go away (Keefe et al 1992).

What does all this tell us about John and Jim? Look through the case studies at the beginning of the chapter again and relate the above information to the cases.

In the clinic

Firstly, don't assume that there will always be a close relationship between clinical examination and factors such as pain report and disability and don't assume that a lack of a relationship demonstrates that the patient is trying to mislead you.

A simple mnemonic developed for the assessment of psychosocial factors in low back pain (Kendall et al 1997) will prompt your thoughts when interviewing a patient.

- A Attitudes and beliefs about the condition
- B Behavior (what they are doing and why they are doing it)
- C Coping (their strategies)
- D Diagnosis (their perceptions of what they have been told and what they actually think themselves)
- E Emotional state (worried, anxious, depressed, frightened)
- F Family (how are their family reacting-being overhelpful, oversolicitous?)
- W Work (what are their perceptions of their ability to return to work, how is their boss reacting to their condition?)

There are a number of simple questionnaires which can be used in clinical practice but it is not clear how the information gained from them can be usefully integrated into treatment. They may be useful to identify those who are struggling and who are likely to need a more careful psychosocial assessment to identify obstacles to recovery. In short, the best source of information is the patient themselves. An interview strategy to be used in association with questionnaires has been developed by Main & Watson (2002) and tested in the clinical setting.

Integrating assessment into practice

There is hardly room in this chapter to cover this immense area but here is a quick tour of the things you can do.

INFORMATION AND REASSURANCE

It seems so obvious that you can only reassure a person once you have found out what they are concerned about. A biopsychosocial assessment tries to determine this. Simple explanations about pain and bland reassurances that things will be all right do not work. One must take time to find out what the patient is worried about, and perform a good clinical examination to demonstrate that you take them seriously and are competent to look for potentially dangerous pathology. Only then will you be able to provide information in a way that is specific to the patient to ensure reassurance. Information should be given in a way commensurate with the patient's understanding of the condition and from their perspective. Well-intentioned reassurance given wrongly can have a disastrous effect.

Providing information about back pain can reduce fear avoidance beliefs but I would not personally advocate providing written information alone without assessing the patient's understanding of it and supporting this with an opportunity to put the advice into practice under supervision in the early stages.

CORRECT MISUNDERSTANDINGS ABOUT PAIN, INJURY AND HARM

Part of the reassurance process is to identify mistaken beliefs about pain and in particular about the link between pain and harm. It is important to help the patient appreciate that an increase in symptoms does not always indicate further damage. An explanation of alternative models of pain physiology has been demonstrated to have some effect (Moseley 2004). Patients who are encouraged to see pain as a complex psychophysiologic problem rather than one purely of structural damage may benefit.

It is important that patients are able to test out new knowledge, Getting them to engage in physical activities which they may be wary of is helpful and specific exercises in a gym setting are one way of doing this. Setting so-called "behavioral experiments" such as performing feared activities or physical tasks helps to challenge the patient's beliefs about the link between activity and harm (Vlaeyen et al 2002b). Successfully performing activities not only reduces fear of activity it also increases self-efficacy, making the patient confident that they can do more. The patient becomes more confident that they can be active despite the pain and that activity will do no harm. Obviously the patient must be informed that increased activity may lead to an increase in discomfort in the short term as a normal process of performing unaccustomed exercise.

GOAL SETTING

As identified above, patients become increasingly depressed if the pain interferes with valued activities. Goal setting – identifying how valued activities can be regained in a systematic way – not only increases self-confidence/ efficacy but successful engagement in such activities reduces the impact of pain and can help improve mood. Goals must be specific, measureable, agreed with the patient, realistic and have a timeframe for achieving them – so-called SMART goals. Goal setting should concentrate on those things the patient values and should include activities they have given up because of the pain (Main et al 2008).

Increase Physical Activity

I think there can be little doubt about the positive effects of physical activity on both physical and mental health. Although there is no direct dose-related response between increased physical activity and reduced disability alone, there is much evidence to support exercise and increasing activity as essential elements in the management of pain (Hayden et al 2005). To date, there is no convincing evidence for one type of exercise over another.

We should not be surprised about this if we consider exercises as mainly a way of engaging people in physical exercise and giving them confidence to be active. The important thing to remember is that any increase in exercise capability should transfer into the achievement of important goals (Main et al 2008); this is the purpose of rehabilitation and I hope physiotherapy remains a *rehabilitation* profession.

Conclusion

Disability due to pain is multifactorial; gone are the days when we thought we could explain disability in terms of pathology or biomechanical restrictions. It is essential that all physiotherapists have an understanding of the factors involved in the development of disability, the ability to identify psychosocial obstacles to recovery and to plan management to overcome them. This does not mean that we should become pseudo-psychologists; we just need to apply some simple psychologic principles to what we do already to remove the obstacles in painful conditions.

Student wisdom

"You should consider reading up on how to talk to your patients and help them through their struggle. You don't need to become a certified psychologist but in practice you will find that those with chronic conditions often have issues that they want to talk about with a health professional (someone like you). Be prepared!" (Anon, USA)

References

Asghari, A., Nicholas, M.K., 2001. Pain self efficacy beliefs and pain behaviour: a prospective study. Pain 94, 85–100.

Bandura, A., 1977. Self-efficacy: toward a unifying theory of behavioral change. Psychol. Rev. 84, 191–215.

Crombez, G., Eccleston, C., Baeyens, F., Van Houdenhove, B., Van Den Broeck, A., 1999. Attention to chronic pain is dependent upon pain-related fear. J. Psychosom. Res. 47, 403–410.

Crombez, G., Van Damme, S., Eccleston, C., 2005. Hypervigilance to pain: an experimental and clinical analysis. Pain 116, 4–7.

Hayden, J.A., Van Tulder, M.W., Tomlinson, G., 2005. Systematic review: strategies for using exercise therapy to improve outcomes in chronic low back pain. Ann. Intern. Med. 142, 776–785.

Keefe, F., Dunsmore, J., 1992. Pain behaviour: concepts and controversies. Pain Forum 1, 92–100.

Keefe, F., Salley, A.N., LeFebvre, J.C., 1992. Coping with pain: conceptual concerns and future references. Pain 51, 131–134.

Kendall, N., Linton, S.J., Main, C.J., 1997. Guide to Assessing Psychosocial Yellow Flags in Acute Low Back Pain: Risk Factors for Long-term Disability and Workloss. Accident Rehabilitation and Compensation Insurance Corporation of New Zealand and the National Health Committee, Ministry of Health, Wellington, New Zealand.

Leeuw, M., Peters, M.L., Wiers, R.W., Vlaeyen, J.W.S., 2007. Measuring fear of movement/(re)injury in chronic low back pain using implicit measures. Cogn. Behav. Ther. 36, 52–64.

Letham, J., Slade, P.D., Troop, J.D.G., Bentley, G., 1983. Outline of a fear-avoidance model of exaggerated pain perception. Behav. Res. Ther. 21, 401–408.

Main, C.J., Watson, P.J., 2002. The distressed and angry low back pain (LBP) patient. In: Gifford, L. (Ed.), Topical Issues in Pain. CNS Press, Falmouth, Cornwall, pp. 175–200.

Main, C., Sullivan, M.J.L., Watson, P.J., 2008. Pain Management: Practical Applications of the Biopsychosocial Perspective in Clinical and Occupational Settings. Churchill Livingstone, Edinburgh.

Morley, S., 2008. Psychology of pain. Br. J. Anaesth. 101, 25–31.

Moseley, G.L., 2004. Evidence for a direct relationship between cognitive and physical change during an education intervention in people with chronic low back pain. Eur. J. Pain. 8, 39–45.

Moseley, G.L., Hodges, P.W., 2006. Reduced variability of postural strategy prevents normalization of motor changes induced by back pain: a risk factor for chronic trouble? Behav. Neurosci. 120, 474–476.

Sullivan, M.J.L., Thorn, B., Haythornthwaite, J.A., 2001. Theoretical perspectives on the relation between catastrophizing and pain. Clin. J. Pain 17 (1), 65–71.

Turner, J.A., Jensen, M.P., Romano, J.M., 2000. Do beliefs, coping and catastrophising independently predict functioning in patients with chronic pain?. Pain 85, 115–125.

Van Damme, S., Crombez, G., Eccleston, C., Roelofs, J., 2004. The role of hypervigilance in the experience of pain. In: Asmundson, G., Vlaeyen, J., Crombez, G. (Eds.) Understanding and Treating Fear of Pain. Oxford University Press, Oxford.

Virchow, R., 1858. Die Cellularpathologie. Hirschwald, Berlin.

Vlaeyen, J.W., Linton, S.J., 2000. Fear-avoidance and its consequences in chronic musculoskeletal pain: a state of the art. Pain 85, 317–332.

Vlaeyen, J.W.S., De Jong, J.R., Onghena, P., Kerckhoffs-Hanssen, M., Kole-Snijders, A.M.J., 2002a. Can pain-related fear be reduced? The application of cognitive-behavioural exposure in vivo. Pain Res. Manag. 7, 144–153.

Vlaeyen, J.W.S., De Jong, J., Geilen, M., Heuts, P., Van Breukelen, G., 2002b. The treatment of fear of movement/(re)injury in chronic low back pain: Further evidence on the effectiveness of exposure in vivo. Clin. J. Pain 18 (4), 251–261.

Waddell, G., 2004. The Back Pain Revolution. Churchill Livingstone, Edinburgh.

Woby, S.R., Roach, N.K., Urmston, M., Watson, P.J., 2007. The relation between cognitive factors and levels of pain and disability in chronic low back pain patients presenting for physiotherapy. Eur. J. Pain 11, 869–877.

Woby, S.R., Roach, N.K., Urmston, M., Watson, P.J., 2008. Outcome following a physiotherapist led intervention for chronic low back pain: the important role of cognitive processes. Physiotherapy 94, 115.

10

Pediatrics
Nick Southorn

- Be a child, it helps!   112
- Childhood diseases   113
- How to assess a child patient   114
- Treatments   117
- Conclusion   118

Studying physiotherapy

This is a very special area of physiotherapy and one that, unfortunately, is delivered at varying levels of quality at university, i.e. it is considered by many clinicians to be somewhat overlooked. That should not diminish your appreciation of this essential topic, however: one should always make an effort to understand childhood-related issues in order to become a competent clinician in any clinical area. The truth is that pediatrics is a challenging topic emotionally, practically, physically and academically.

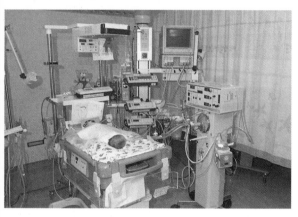

Fig. 10.1 Emotional challenges range from seeing little babies on the neonatal intensive care unit to much older children with incapacitating illnesses. (Reproduced from Pryor & Prasad 2002, with kind permission from Elsevier.)

Be a child, it helps!

The first thing to remember is that children are not merely "little adults." They respond differently in almost every way to almost everything you do. It all begins at the first meeting. Stay with me here: shrink down to about 4 feet tall – doesn't everything seem so much more imposing all of a sudden? Maybe even a little scary ... Now walk about your neighborhood at this height: people going about their business as normal, barely noticing you as they rush on by. Now imagine you are attending a hospital appointment because someone noticed you aren't quite the same as other kids your age ... and a strange adult bursts into the room and begins talking. Now imagine you are the adult walking into that room – what do you do? Even if they have seen many clinicians before you, when you first meet that child you *must* make a good impression, gain trust and settle nerves (that also applies to the parent/carer attending with the child).

How you treat children also differs from adults. Although in adults we attempt to encourage self-efficacy combined with manual techniques, a lot of treatment is "passive" (i.e. the therapist does the work) as that appears to do the trick. It is well established that many childhood conditions, such as cerebral palsy, may require more intensive treatment and as therapy contact may be limited, we must alter our treatment pattern. In each year there are approximately 8736 hours and even if a patient receives physiotherapy for an hour a day through the working week (which is considerably more than the majority actually get), they will only have 260 therapy hours per year! So what do we do? Two things: educate the parents/carers to help perform the exercises and continue to monitor to ensure they are doing it correctly and issue progression if necessary; and if the child is old enough/has adequate cognitive skills, teach the exercises in a fun and enjoyable way to the child. This goes a long way to give ownership of the treatment to the child and perhaps decrease the dependence on health professionals.

I'm going to ask you to use your imagination again now. You are working full time (not as a health professional, as something else) to pay the bills as we all do throughout our life. You also have a 2-year-old child in whom the health visitor has spotted suspicious symptoms and so has referred you to a pediatrician. You have no idea what the implications are, what the possible conditions are, etc.; you just know that your precious child could be seriously ill. You attend the appointment on Monday afternoon, taking time off work, and the consultant refers your child for further assessment/investigations which could include speech and language therapy, occupational therapy, physiotherapy, blood tests, audiologist, optician, dietician, etc. All of these appointments you *have* to attend for the sake of your child's health. Children are usually seen by myriad professionals, for good reason, but the burden on the parents is immense – please consider this. Many centers now employ an integrated appointment to reduce the number of visits but you could still ease the load slightly by encouraging home treatment by the parents/carers or synchronizing physio appointments with other health providers.

How did you develop?

Learning about pediatrics is a case of knowing about normal child development. Of course, there is the obvious motor and psychologic development that is used to define how a child is doing in relation to the norm (such as absence of head lag when pulled to sit at 4 months, sitting unsupported at 6 months, etc.) and you should become familiar with these but what about anatomic and physiologic differences in terms of cardiorespiratory, bone, nerves, etc.? Knowing about the "normal" child will allow you to determine a degree of severity/prognosis for any pathology. A great book that remains *the* guide on development is *From birth to five years* by Mary D Sheridan: Sheridan, Sharma & Frost (1997).

Childhood diseases

There are many syndromes and diseases that you will come across in pediatrics. You should begin with the more common conditions and develop a solid knowledge of these, such as cerebral palsy (CP), cystic fibrosis (CF), Down's syndrome, spina bifida, and a handful of degenerative muscular conditions such as Duchenne muscular dystrophy. Some conditions not seen by the adult physiotherapist 20 or 30 years ago are making the transition to adult care as more and more patients with these conditions make it to their second and third decades of life and therefore may arrive on your patient list even if you are not a pediatric physiotherapist. Alternatively, someone you are treating has a child with one of these conditions; would you know instinctively how the child's care is affected by your patient's condition? The answer – learn about them! The exact pathophysiologic processes of a lot of these conditions (as with many neurologic conditions) can be vague at times so a "physiologic leap of faith" is needed but only if the safety net of your existing knowledge of the healthy body is in place – get the basics down first!

How to assess a child patient

I recommend two books relating to the general physiotherapy of children, including great sections on assessment: *Physical management in neurological rehabilitation* (Stokes 2004) and *Physiotherapy for respiratory and cardiac problems* (Pryor & Prasad 2002). The assessment is immensely important in pediatric physiotherapy (mostly in relation to neurologic conditions) as it forms part of a bigger picture. As such, you *must* dedicate time to understanding the principles of assessment.

You will need to create a concise and conclusive report that is used to either facilitate or confirm a diagnosis. This is very different from, say, orthopedics in which you assess and diagnose freely – in pediatrics everyone involved has an opinion that has implications for their colleagues, the patient and their parents/carers. Things that you should consider when learning how to perform a subjective assessment include the following (you are expected to research and understand the implications of each of these).

Subjective assessment

HISTORY

- Did the child reach full term?*
- Were there any birth complications?*
- Have there been any significant incidents/trauma that may explain the symptoms?*
- Other relevant history of present condition (nature, severity, frequency) – remember the usual HPC questions such as aggravating/easing factors, impact upon daily life, sleeping patterns, etc.
- Medical/surgical history – including dates and whether problems persist.
- Treatments/investigations – results.
- Drug history – including dose and any difficulties taking them.

PROBLEMS

- What, in the patient/parent/carer's words, are the main problems? Problem-orientated assessments will give you a good idea of the perceived problem and allow you to assess the patient's/carer's understanding of the condition and whether they have a realistic grasp of the prognosis.

- This may even be an appropriate time to discuss potential barriers to full functional rehabilitation, i.e. do they live in rented accommodation and therefore can't have adaptations? Can the family attend rehabilitation sessions regularly (cost, transport, time)? Are the parents/carers willing to take on the role of therapist if need be?

You may have guessed that the initial assessment is time consuming. It also demands a certain tactfulness, hence the (*) above. Get what you can from the existing medical records: this will allow you to skip over potentially painful memories such as traumatic childbirth, accidents involving children, etc.

Objective assessment

The objective assessment on initial contact is also quite lengthy as you need to establish a definite objective marker that will enable you to establish goals and evaluate any progress. Without going into too much detail, it is very much worth studying the following.

JOINT FUNCTION

- ROM
- Quality of movement
- Type of end feel
- Reflexes – is there one? Is it rather brisk? What are the implications of this?

MUSCLES

- Strength – the Medical Research Council scale below (MRC 1978) is used in the UK.
    0 No activity
    1 Minimal contraction but insufficient to move joint
    2 Movement of joint with gravity counterbalanced
    3 Muscle activity able to move joint against gravity but not against resistance
    4 Activity able to move joint against moderate resistance (but not to previous levels)
    5 Normal activity
- Tone – define tone, spasticity and rigidity. What can cause high and low tone? What scale is used to measure tone?
- Bulk – atrophy/distribution (i.e. has there been a rupture?)/hypertrophy? What could the implications of increased muscle mass be? Is it true muscle bulk or pseudohypertrophy?

SENSATION

- Hot/cold
- Sharp/soft

- Graphesthesia
- Proprioception

GAIT AND BALANCE

- Learn how to observe normal gait properly before attempting pathologic gait.
- The Berg Balance Scale (Berg et al 1992) below uses a score of s4 for each of the dimensions (1 = poor attempt at task and 4 = success at task).

  1. Sit to stand
  2. Stand unsupported
  3. Sit unsupported
  4. Stand to sit
  5. Transfers
  6. Stand with eyes closed
  7. Stand with feet together
  8. Reach forward with arms stretched forward
  9. Pick up object on the floor
  10. Turn to look behind
  11. Turn on the spot 360°
  12. Placing alternate feet on a step
  13. Stand with one foot in front of the other
  14. Stand on one foot

FUNCTIONAL ACTIVITY

- Are there adaptations/compensations?
- Is it safe and effective?
- Use the *International classification of functioning, disability and health* (WHO 2001)

This is a quick overview of the things you should learn about. All of this may seem quite familiar; so it should, it does mirror an adult but with one major difference: how on earth are you going to get all of this information from a child? How can you make it fun without compromising the results? Will you keep the child's concentration long enough? What if there is a communication barrier (it is likely)?

Remember that you need to know about the diagnostics too. Electro-diagnostic tests such as electroencephalography (EEG) and nerve conduction studies may help you form a clinical impression. Imaging such as computed tomography (CT), magnetic resonance imaging (MRI), angiography, and positron emission tomography (PET) are used regularly and should form part of your study. Other investigations that you will come across are: spirometry; arterial blood gasses (ABGs), although in the child you may only see these in the neonatal and intensive care setting, otherwise the capillary blood gasses may be used; electrocardiograph (ECG); exercise testing, which is used extensively in children (and adults) with respiratory conditions such as cystic fibrosis as an objective marker and an additional form of exercise.

Treatments

When an onlooker catches a glimpse of a pediatric physiotherapist treating a child, they, quite rightly, conclude that it is just playing about. Of course it is – how else are you going to get a child to contract their tibialis anterior muscle without pretending that the toy crocodile is going to nibble their toes if they don't!

Your job is to engage with the child; if they are 4 years old then play with 4-year-old type stuff like train sets, dolls' houses, toy vacuum cleaners and other toddler toys. If they are 10 then play with a football, skipping rope, hop-scotch (Himmel und Holle/Puz/Kith-Kith/Potsy) and other young person games. The challenge is making it *therapeutic* play, i.e. playing so that the activity forms a therapeutic exercise. For example, development of core muscles can be enhanced with bridging while a train is passed underneath the body ("*How many times can the train pass under?*") or playing on an inflatable physio ball (Swiss ball/gym ball), playing catch, etc. Treating children will challenge your initiative to the limits and beyond; you will constantly be amazed at how you can be so creative and how they can bring out the best in you. Have a think about some activities children do and what muscles are being worked or how out of breath they get and link it to a pathology you know. It's a great way of lateral thinking.

Respiratory treatments can be less subtle as some are overtly a treatment; percussion, for example, is hard to disguise as play. However, these children are usually well aware of their condition and the importance of treatment. Sport is usually employed for respiratory treatments as it has the effect of enhancing the cardiorespiratory function and creating a situation in which any secretions are well mobilized and eventually self-expectorated.

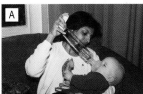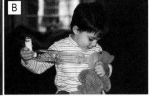

Fig. 10.2 Treating children respiratory management and making it fun is a real test of imagination. Babies sometimes just need a rattle to play with (A) whereas older children may want to engage more with the treatment and administer bronchodilators to teddy (B). (Reproduced from Pryor & Prasad 2002, with kind permission from Elsevier.)

In the course of a long-standing physical condition, it will become apparent to the patient that they will not make a full recovery or even get any better. This is typical for the muscular dystrophy and cerebral palsy children and your answer had better be good. As a student, it is worth thinking about why you are treating someone who isn't going to get better. Just have a think about cerebral palsy for a moment. Sure, it is a nonprogressive disorder but if the condition is the same at the age of 15 as it was at 3, just think about how much more difficult sustaining controlled movement is now the limbs are longer, the body is much bigger and heavier, etc. One is also more body aware at 15 – how will that affect the patient? How about the Duchenne muscular dystrophy boy who knows he will probably be dead in 10 years' time?

It's all about maintaining quality of life and current function for as long as possible. It should never be underestimated how much difference it makes for the patient/carer/parent if they can perhaps stand and use a handrail to hold themselves up for 5 minutes while they are changed. That function can be easily lost when motivation is low and rehab is poor and it is difficult to get back. So when you hear of a "nondegenerative" condition, try to put it into context.

Conclusion

Working with children is the most exciting and engaging area of physiotherapy. It is hard work to begin with – learning how to communicate with children of all abilities and how to get the best out of them, usually by bribing them with stickers! However, it can also be one of the most rewarding so it is all well worth the effort. As I identified at the beginning of this chapter, pediatrics is largely under-represented at university and some people are actually arranging pediatric placements in addition to their university ones if one is not offered by the institution. We hope that the profession one day recognizes pediatrics as a core topic and offers it more time on the syllabus.

The words "have fun" are a key feature of this book; when you are learning about and working with children, they don't even have to be said – you just will!

References

Berg, K.O., Maki, B.E., Williams, J.I., et al., 1992. Clinical and laboratory measures of postural balance in an elderly population. Arch. Phys. Med. Rehabil. 73, 1073–1080.

Medical Research Council, 1978. Aids to the Examination of the Peripheral Nervous System. Baillière Tindall, Eastbourne.

Pryor, J.A., Prasad, S.A., 2002. Physiotherapy for Respiratory and Cardiac Problems: Adults and Paediatrics, third ed. Churchill Livingstone, Edinburgh.

Sheridan, M., Sharma, A., Frost, M., 1997. From Birth to Five Years, seconnd ed. Routledge, London.

Stokes, J., 2004. Physical Management in Neurological Rehabilitation, second ed. Mosby Elsevier, Edinburgh.

World Health Organization 2001 International classification of functioning, disability and health. Available at: www.who.int/classification/icf

11

Clinical placement
Nick Southorn

- How to prepare 120
- What you need to know before you get there 122
- Uniform etiquette 122
- What you need to know when you get there 126
- The learning agreement 128
- Marking criteria 128
- The role of the clinical educator 130
- The role of the academic tutor 131
- Conclusion 131

Studying physiotherapy

Let's get to the point – nerves! It is perfectly normal to be nervous before your first placement. Clinical educators know this and should allow for this. Don't panic – they don't expect you to arrive, pick up a patient list and begin treating!

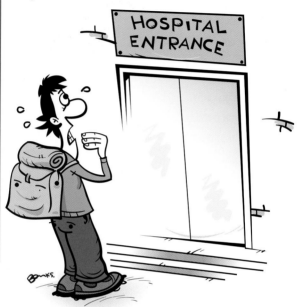

Fig. 11.1 Don't panic! They don't expect you to just start treating patients – you are a student, remember.

Clinical placements are the most taxing part of your physiotherapy degree for a number of reasons: you are expected to put into practice what, in theory, you know from book reading, you will just be settling into your placement and you then have to rotate or it comes to an end, you are constantly "the student" and can feel as though you get under people's feet, and you are generally shattered all the time! However, placements are the most valuable part too. You will be shocked at exactly how much you will learn from educators of all professions and patients from all backgrounds. Placements will open your eyes to the practicalities of being a physiotherapist and give you pure insight that you can't read about in books. It is often said that only in clinical placements can you decide what area of this diverse profession you would like to work in. If you take one thing from this chapter, it should be that you should enjoy your placements and learn from them.

How to prepare

The best way you can prepare is to be well informed as to the nature of the placement. Don't try to guess as you may find that you have missed the mark entirely. To do this, you should find out who is your clinical educator and give them a ring. Your university placement organizer will happily give you the information you need to contact them. Actually, most expect you to do this: it shows that you are a confident and conscientious student and is an easy way to make a good first impression. It helps if you have everything you need to say written down clearly in front of you; there is nothing worse than being asked your phone number and forgetting it! Make sure they know what placement number you are on, eliminating *any* possibility of error on their part. For example, if this is your first placement and they are expecting a third placement student, they are going to expect much more from you. This does happen and it is not a good start to placement number one! See below under "What you need to know before you get there" for starter questions. Although you have a list of questions written down, you should remember that you are having a conversation, i.e. don't be too rigid in your structure, allow the conversation to flow and let them ask questions along the way too.

Usually your first placement, regardless of the area you are in, will be a test of your assessment technique. My most valuable bit of advice to you is to learn how to assess a patient thoroughly. This may sound easy but believe me, it isn't as simple as that. A comprehensive assessment includes the impact of the pathology not only on the physical aspect but also on the functional (Activities of Daily Living) and the psychologic. Also, you need to understand the consequences of the answers you get quite quickly, e.g. if the patient has kidney failure, what implications are there for the musculoskeletal system or the blood pressure? If a patient presents with back pain and on assessment it appears has saddle anesthesia and urinary incontinence, what do you do? These are all very important and, luckily, usually specific to a particular clinical area.

When you do find out what type of patient you are likely to see, it is imperative that you learn how to assess them as this will save you a lot of time and earn you lots of brownie points! You need to discover the medications the patient is taking and for what (e.g. a beta-blocker could be for migraines as well as for hypertension) and diurnal patterns, etc. Each bit of information is important in making a diagnosis. As for the objective assessment, look at everything that has been done – blood tests, X-rays and so on – to give yourself a full picture. You won't be expected to develop a completely clinically reasoned explanation for the findings immediately but if you have a basic understanding for each individual test, that is a good start. It is usually a good idea to get a group of friends together and use each other as patients; it's a much better way of learning than auscultation on a pillow! If you are playing the part of the patient then you also get to describe how your colleagues are doing. Always remember that in the "role play" setting as well as the clinical setting, you should always *gain informed consent* from your friend/the patient.

You should also prepare your social life too. Unlike other university students, you are about to have no time at all! Clinical placements are all-encompassing and are severely detrimental to your social life. You get up early, have about 30 minutes for lunch (during which you are reading) and by the time you get home you are completely knackered but still have more reading to do! It is therefore important to *always* make time to see friends and family at weekends, evenings, etc. You have to switch off and give your poor brain a rest otherwise you will not last the duration. Make sure that someone on your course prepares a "pre-placement party" to blow off steam before you all disappear.

What you need to know before you get there

OK, so you are about to ring your clinical educator: what are you going to ask? Here are a few generic questions that may help you.

- What time do you want me to arrive? Take this time and make it 15 mins earlier. Being late is a big no-no.
- Do you have any specific uniform guidelines, i.e. shirt, tie and trousers or tracksuit?
- Are there any changing facilities available in the unit/hospital? Also ask about lockers/secure storage of kit.
- What type of patients do you see?
  - Conditions?
  - Length of stay?
  - Typical rehab/treatment (physio/medical/others)?
  - Other professional members involvement (assistants/OTs/podiatrists/ doctors, etc.)
- Do I need any specialist equipment?
  - Goniometer
  - Stethoscope
  - Swimming trunks/costume, etc.
- Should I do any preparatory reading on the area? You should always do some but they may have some specific ideas as to what they expect you to read.
- Are there any information leaflets that I can have about the area? Each area usually has written information available for students.

You are obliged to ensure that all entries into medical records are countersigned by a qualified member of staff. Remember that no matter how good you are, you are a student and therefore should never be in a position where you feel unsupported by qualified staff. If you don't know the answer to something, the *worst* thing to do is keep it quiet. Now is your opportunity to ask questions and be sure of the answers. Always be safe and just think ahead of time about what you are about to do and you'll be just fine. You will naturally learn where the fine line is between being independent and autonomous, and dangerous practice – you will also *always* strive never to cross that line.

Uniform etiquette

You may not have used it since your interview but now the iron has to re-emerge. Not all physio students follow this principle but having an ironed uniform makes the world of difference. Your uniform should be clean and tidy as once you walk into the hospital or clinic, you become a representative of your school, your profession and yourself; you should strive to make a good impression at all times. It is always a good idea to travel to your placement in your civilian clothes and change once you are there, even if you are expected to wear a shirt and tie. Hospital infection is a major issue and one that should be taken very seriously by everyone, from visiting relatives to the

chief executive. Ensure that a name badge is seen at all times as per the local

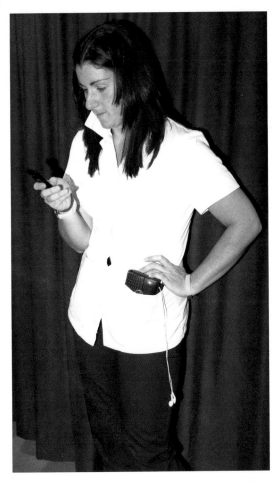

Fig. 11.2 Apearances are everything! Don't let yourself down by looking rough! (A) A student who fills their pockets with gadgetry and texts is asking for trouble. (B) The student who irons their uniform and looks smart and interested will go far! (C) This is a common sight in the staff room at lunch but don't forget that even at lunch time, you are still on the clock. Your clinical educator has to be impressed too.

policy. Hair should be tied up if necessary – this is something that all physios should adhere to; it only needs to happen once for you to know why. I'm told that having a patient swing from a pony tail when they are heading floorwards is not a nice experience! You will have found out what the uniform policy is before you get there if you are organized and that is what they will expect from

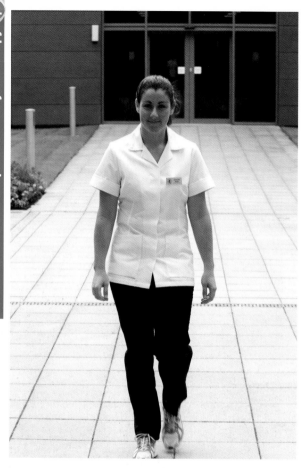

Fig. 11.2 (Continued)

you. If you try to "bend" the rules by wearing something that resembles the uniform but isn't, then you can expect a stern talking to.

Your student badge should be well looked after. Don't lose it as it is a nightmare to replace and your clinical educator will rightly question your organizational skills. I can also advise that the washing machine is no place for your name badge either! In hospitals, health clinics, schools, i.e. anywhere that you will be placed, it is vital that you can identify yourself with appropriate identification and justify being there. I would expect somone not wearing a name badge to be escorted from the premises.

If jewelery can be avoided, please do so: these things are a magnet for infection, for one thing, and if your patient has allergies to metals, has a

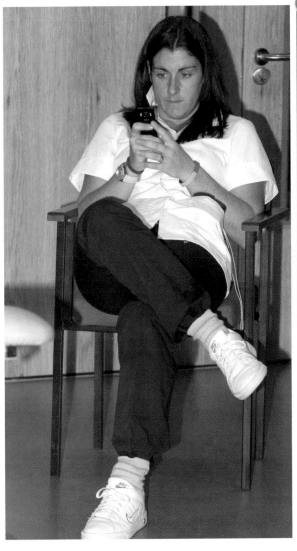

Fig. 11.2 (Continued)

condition or is taking any medication that affects their skin, you may cause some serious damage. Be considerate and remove rings, watches and so on.

Don't take your mobile onto the ward, it's just rank bad manners. You are there to do your job for the patients, to impress the educator and to learn; Sod's Law dictates that you will forget to turn the ringer off and someone will call you while you are consulting. It also sets a bad example to the patients: mobile phones are discouraged in hospitals and that should include staff. On that note, you should only take what you need with you to the clinical area, i.e. a couple of pens, notepad, pocket book, etc. No iPod, wallet, keys, chocolate bars or lipstick. All, especially keys, can cause potential harm to the patient and can be easily lost.

As mentioned before, a notepad is an essential bit of kit. It can be used for things like phone numbers, names, door codes, etc. and, more importantly, any clinical tips that the educator throws your way. Just a note on door codes: disguise them as something else, if not for your sake then for the sake of everyone else! A vital part of any student's uniform is *The physiotherapist's pocket book* (Kenyon & Kenyon 2009). It is a quick reference guide to being a clinician and is easily cleaned with an alcoholic wipe. Any student or junior physiotherapist can be identified by the pink book in their pocket.

Your uniform should be clean and dry. Obvious? You'd have thought so! Washing your kit at 60°C will kill micro-organisms but if you use the right detergent, you can wash at 40°C to have the same effect and be slightly more eco-friendly. Having your kit washed every 2 days is usually acceptable unless an obvious reason for an earlier wash is arises (you'll know when it happens). However, local rules rule! Regardless of what you read elsewhere, it is what you are told by your clinical educator/staff member that is important – what they say goes.

Clinical educators have said that what is worse than a dirty uniform is one that has obviously dried while in a ball in the wash basket! They give off a musky smell that isn't pleasant so hang your uniform to dry for the sake of social etiquette!

What you need to know when you get there

When you arrive you will get a guided tour of the premises. It is all too easy to follow the educator around, nodding politely, wondering when the cool bits start, but remember that you will be expected to recall this information if anything happens.

WHAT TO DO IN A FIRE

- What does the alarm sound like?
- When is alarm test date (usually once a week)?
- Emergency exits?
- Who is the Fire Officer?
- What is the number to call in case of fire?
- Where are the fire blankets and extinguishers?
- Where is the assembly point?
- If in a ward, what happens to the patients?

IF YOU WITNESS A CARDIAC ARREST/COLLAPSE/ACCIDENT, ETC.

- Who is trained to take this on (you will have basic training but there will be an advanced team about)?
- How can the crash team be contacted?
- If you are unsure as to your basic training or you are in a high-risk area, i.e. critical care, please ask for additional or refresher training.

WHO'S WHO?

- Reception/clerical team.
- Other professionals, especially those not in a uniform.
- People you will be working with. It is excruciatingly embarrassing to forget the names of the people who are training you so take a notebook and note their names.

PHONE ETIQUETTE

- How does one answer the phone in this department?
- Should you even answer the phone?

PHONE NUMBERS

- If you are unable to attend for whatever reason or you are delayed on a house call, who you gonna call?

BREAK/LUNCH TIMES

- Don't be too keen to ask this question!

LIBRARY/COMPUTER ACCESS

- For educational (revising, researching) and clinical needs (X-rays, results).

LOCATION OF ANY EMERGENCY/SPECIALIST EQUIPMENT

- Crash trolley, suction kit, phones, etc. in case you are told to get them.
- Crutches, frames, therapeutic equipment. It is just as important to know the whereabouts of these too!

I'm sure that other questions will become apparent during your introduction to the unit. You should be interested in the location of the health and safety manual and the accident book too. Once you have all this information, you can begin to relax into your placement.

Questions specific to the area you work in should come naturally to you. It is sometimes wise to ask questions even if you know the answer. Showing an extended interest in your placement will do wonders in making that first impression. Ask yourself these questions.

- Do you know the most common pathology of the department?
- Who is the most senior clinician here?

- What specialties are covered here?
- Are there any maximum treatment periods or targets that clinicians have to meet?
- Are there any protocols (usually in orthopedics) to follow?

These are just a few guidance questions to get you started!

The learning agreement

The learning agreement is a "contract" between the educator and the student. This is where you get to put down in words exactly what you want from the placement. These are your demands! Do be specific with these in terms of how you will achieve them and exactly what it is you want to achieve. Don't include too many as they will no longer be achievable. Make them realistic, i.e. "to be competent in acupuncture for back pain" may be pushing it a little but "to learn the principles of Western acupuncture for lower back pain" is more likely to be achieved. In simple terms, they have to be like any other goals that you may set for your patients: SMART (see p.000).

It is wise to begin this process within the first few days of the placement. Involve the clinical educator from the start and ensure that they are clear as to what it is you want. Do make the contract a fluid and dynamic document, though; it should never be set in stone and you should *always* carry a copy about with you to refer to whenever possible. Make adjustments to it all the time as it shows you are adapting to the environment. If you have what you'd consider to be a more outrageous addition to the agreement that you would like to experience, you should never be afraid to ask your educator. All placements are a real opportunity for you to discover physiotherapy. If you would like to experience time with an acupuncturist or spend a day in surgery watching a relevant operation then just ask. It is that simple. Your physiotherapy degree should be seen as an opportunity to really explore the profession as you may not get another chance!

Once you have some clear idea of what you are aiming for, remember that you should be taking the initiative when it comes to completing it. Don't rely on the clinical educator to spoon feed you all the time.

Once you have completed your learning agreement tasks you may wish to print off a final copy of your achievements throughout the placements and have your clinical educator sign it as a nice addition to your portfolio.

Marking criteria

The marking criteria will vary significantly depending on what university you are studying at. You need to access this information and scan through it before you start your placement. Some universities use a set time to go through this in a structured way and give you the opportunity to play at being a clinical educator to mark a fictional student. This is a valuable exercise that should be encouraged; even if your university doesn't offer this exercise, it is easily done with friends.

When you get the criteria you should get to know them quite well and understand what each of the definitions are within the marking guidelines. If you don't know and understand this, how will you know what you are working towards? Remember that if you are doing something very clever that will help you get good marks, let the clinical educator know what you are doing. It's no good if only you know about it! Also, demonstrate your clinical reasoning skills by evolving your questioning skills. For example, you may start by presenting your findings from your assessment followed by "What should I do now?" then, once you are more clinically aware, "I think that I should do this," eventually leading to "This is what I have found; this is what I intend to do." If you are wrong then, fine, you need to work on your clinical reasoning and that's a fair comment. However, if you are right they have no choice but to give you good marks. The moral of this is to sell yourself. Purposefully let the clinical educator see the things that you do and ask if you are unsure about a technique.

FAQs on placements

Q. What should I do if I'm finding I don't have enough time to write up my notes?

A. Discuss this with your clinical educator and ask for an increased time allowance for note writing. Produce your own checklist of things that should be documented in the notes and possibly find some "gold standard" examples from other physios to use as a reference.

Q. What do I do if I realize I've given a patient some incorrect advice after they have been discharged?

A. Don't panic! Tell your clinical educator. Locate the patient's details and telephone number. Ring them at home if appropriate. Document your phone call and the subsequent advice. Remember, physiotherapists are in a position of responsibility. It is of the utmost importance to *always* be honest, open and do your best by the patient.

Q. What if the hours are clashing with work/family commitments?

A. Speak to your clinical educator. They are trained to deal with this and will come to some agreement with you regarding shifting hours about. It is important to remember that "just putting up with it" will never do. Ultimately if your potential can't be realized because of additional stresses, it is not only you who suffers: your clinical educator and your patients are all influenced by your actions. Use your clinical educator – they are there to help you get the most from your placement.

You will do well to remember that you should always be honest with yourself and be open to constructive criticism. If you truly believe that the clinical educator is marking you unfairly then you are well within your rights to ask them to justify it. However, it has been known that the student's marks have suffered due to a conflict of personality. This should *never* happen, ever. Any differences should be aired and, as a professional, you should be open and receptive to others' opinions, as they should be with you. If a genuine grievance is noted and your marks suffer as a consequence, you should always seek the advice of your academic tutor.

The role of the clinical educator

It is important that you understand the academic role of everyone involved in your placement. This will allow smooth running to be maintained if any issues arise. In this section, I will also discuss the use of mentors and other clinical auxiliaries that you may come across through your placement.

The clinical educator is your main contact and is the clinical manager of your placement. Your clinical educator may be a relatively junior physical therapist and so will have to report back to his or her senior on your progress. This is to meet their training needs and nothing to worry you at all. Whatever the level of your clinical educator, they will have responsibilities beyond those of your placement. You will do well to respect that they are, primarily, clinicians with a caseload and are taking the time with you to benefit the profession. However, they do have a responsibility to you and if regular fenced-off time with you is being missed for whatever reason, you must mention it. It is not acceptable for you to miss out on this valuable experience because of the workload of the educator.

So, what do they do for you? Well, this is a hard area to generalize on as the involvement will vary considerably from person to person. Generally speaking, their involvement with your patient contact should be quite significant to begin with, eventually decreasing as you become more experienced. A good and organized clinical educator will have:

- informed other staff from all professions that you are expected and where you are in your learning
- a plan of training for the formative days/weeks of your placement
- a comprehensive induction that should result in you feeling confident around the department
- ring-fenced protected time for you to study that is not affected by anything within reason
- a good idea as to what your learning agreement should consist of
- a reasonable level of understanding of your past training (however, as most educators cover a number of different physio schools, this may be difficult)
- the details of your academic tutor, including the proposed visiting date
- a detailed knowledge of your marking criteria.

A good clinical educator will also seek to accommodate your learning style and provide a suitable platform for you to learn. This is a two-way street, though, and this can only be accomplished by communication. Don't be afraid to tell your clinical educator what you want. Also, a good educator will encourage autonomous practice and learning; this is part of being a professional and should be nurtured from early on. A bad clinical educator will insist that you do exactly what they do in exactly the same way. This failure to recognize someone's individuality can be of huge detriment to what would normally be a great placement. This is a scenario that should be discussed with your academic tutor.

The role of the academic tutor

Your academic tutor can be described as a nonclinical manager of your placement. They provide the unsung support from afar and, hopefully, provide you with a feeling of back-up if it is needed. Given the scenario mentioned before with the clashing personalities, this is exactly the area that the academic tutor specializes in. However, if they seem "stand-offish" that is purely because they are allowing you the opportunity to deal with the situation yourself. On reflection, you will feel a greater sense of achievement for it. Nonetheless, if you feel that a situation is out of your comfort zone you may insist that the academic tutor steps in and develops a solution. It will mostly be a compromise but an agreement will eventually be reached.

They can offer guidance and support that can develop your placement into the best it can be. Typically you will see your academic tutor once every 2–3 weeks but they will attend as often as you like. *You* are their priority. They will appreciate being involved in the goal setting for your placement; they know what you have and haven't done at university and therefore are ideally placed to help you with this.

They will also chat to your clinical educator – it is a time for them to discuss how good you are and how far they can push you.

Above all, academic tutor visits offer a legitimate reason to have some time off from your placement and have a chat!

Conclusion

So, go forth and be nervous! It will all become natural soon enough and you will wonder what all the fuss was about. I hope that this chapter has given you a bit more insight into what you can expect from clinical education and as a result you will enter your placement with your eyes wide open and get the most from it. Remember the embarrassing moments, the good, the bad – they make you who you are. No matter what happens, you always have the back-up of your academic tutor and your friends. Use them well and enjoy the time off from university. Before you know it, you will be back sitting exams.

Student wisdom

"Remember to create a portfolio and record evidence (reflective writing, personal development plans, placement objectives, etc.) as soon as you can as it will help you immensely in the long term in terms of applying for jobs and continuing the process as a clinician." (Suzanne Temple, Nottingham, UK)

"Be honest with yourself and your educator while on placement. If you feel you need more or less support, tell someone. Worrying about not knowing something you think you should know will only make the situation worse and it could affect your performance, final grade and (worse case scenario) employability." (Ronan Donohoe, Clonee, Ireland)

"Having assessed my patient I determined he had reduced thoracic mobility and as such prescribed extension exercises – he complained of chest problems and found the exercises difficult. Having discussed this with my clinical educator I explained that the extensions would also help with the chest pain – he soon discovered that he was capable of the exercises and soon improved! Always describe exercises in terms of the patient's complaint rather than what you find on examination (and make good use of your educator)." (Verena Bensaddik-Brunner, Geneva, Switzerland)

References

Kenyon, J., Kenyon, K., 2009. The Physiotherapist's Pocket Book, second ed. Churchill Livingstone, Edinburgh.

Section 3
The final stretch

The final section now signifies your transition from student to professional practitioner. You should feel that, by now, you have adequate knowledge relating to the human body and need to concentrate on ways to apply this knowledge in a professional and mature way, even thinking about how you can contribute to the physiotherapy/medical knowledge base by research. All the while keeping in mind that you need to spend more time with friends as the university days come to an end.

Chapter 12 **Clinical audit and research** 135

Chapter 13 **The degree continues** 143

Chapter 14 **You think it's all over …** 157

Clinical audit and research

Herbert Thurston

- Clinical audit   136
- Research   136

The final stretch

Students studying for a degree in healthcare can expect to learn about clinical audit and research at an early stage in their course. Some consider that clinical audit is a form of research and indeed, the two are related, often with one feeding into the other. However, despite this relationship there are important differences between clinical audit and research. Clinical audit is concerned with providing the best care whereas the motivation for research is the generation of new knowledge. Also, there are many differences in the investigation processes involved.

Clinical audit

- Ascertains whether an existing service reaches a predetermined standard.
- Involves interrogation of records or completing a questionnaire.
- Research ethics committee review is not required.

Research

- Often is deductive and concerned with critical testing.
- May involve a new treatment, additional therapy and investigations.
- May involve random allocation to treatment or control groups.
- Requires research ethics committee review and approval.

Clinical audit

Defined in a government White Paper as "the systematic, critical analysis of the quality of medical care, including the procedures used for diagnosis and treatment, the use of resources and the resulting outcome and quality of life for the patient," audit was introduced into the NHS in 1989. Initially aimed at doctors, subsequently the Department of Health encouraged other healthcare professionals to undertake audit and in 1993 established multiprofessional audit. This led to a change in title to clinical audit, which involves all healthcare professionals.

THE CLINICAL AUDIT CYCLE

- Setting care standards (based on guidelines and expert opinion).
- Preparing a questionnaire for data collection to assess current practice.
- Collation and analysis of data.
- Presenting a summary with recommendations to healthcare providers.
- After an interval, repeating the audit process.
- The latter step of the audit cycle is commonly termed "closing the loop."

Research

Many undergraduate students feel that research is not for them and a common definition describing research as "an endeavor to discover new or collate old facts by scientific study of a subject or by a course of critical investigation" does nothing to change this view. However, research is not the exclusive preserve of academics and laboratory scientists; any student with a good idea should be able to frame a question and undertake a research project.

For example, in 1921 a young medical practitioner called Frederick Banting went to the Department of Physiology in the University of Toronto with a new idea about diabetes mellitus which lead to the discovery of insulin in 1922. At that time, it was well known that the pancreas was vital for the maintenance of a normal blood sugar level and removing the pancreas resulted in experimentally induced diabetes mellitus. However, despite many years of research in the best centers in the world, it had not been possible to extract the active hormone from pancreatic tissue. Banting was of the opinion that digestive enzymes became activated in the pancreas, destroying the hormone during the extraction process. Previous studies had shown that pancreatic duct ligation resulted in pancreatic atrophy but diabetes mellitus did not develop. This knowledge allowed Banting to make a pancreatic preparation from which insulin could be isolated. Clearly, a surgical approach would not permit insulin production on a large scale but Banting's experiments led to the development of laboratory techniques for isolating insulin from the pancreas of pigs and cows. The rest, as they say, is history. Students will be interested to learn that Frederick Banting, who graduated from the University of Toronto, had little or no research experience and his co-worker was still a medical student at the time they discovered insulin. The medical student, Charles Herbert Best, subsequently went on to become Professor of Physiology and Head of the Banting Best Medical Research Institute at Toronto University.

Types of research

Clinical research can be broadly divided into *observational research*, concerned with collecting data from individual patients or groups of patients, and *experimental research* which involves comparing the response of groups of patients to different treatment interventions.

OBSERVATIONAL RESEARCH

Studies involving the collection of numeric data, e.g. body weight and height, blood pressure, pulse rate, the range of joint movement, etc. are called *quantitative research*. This form of research involves the use of tools or questionnaires and provides numeric data which can be subjected to statistical analysis. This can also be used to test hypotheses.

Studies concerned with recording patients' experiences, thoughts, feelings and perceptions are called *qualitative research* and usually do not provide numeric data. Such approaches are quite subjective because the researcher collects and interprets descriptive information obtained at interview. An interview may be *structured*, where each participant is asked to provide answers to a set of fixed questionnaires, or *semi-structured*, using a set of open-ended questionnaires. Occasionally, *unstructured* interviews are conducted, allowing the participant to talk about their concerns rather than answering the interviewer's questions. But inevitably, information from an unstructured interview is more difficult to interpret.

Despite some concerns that qualitative research can be subjective because the researcher has a central role in the conduct of the interview and interpreting participants' responses to questions, this approach is well accepted and makes important contributions to patient care.

For example, in the early days of cardiac rehabilitation, the coronary unit at the Leicester Royal Infirmary set up a study to discover whether patients found participating in the cardiac rehabilitation program provided by a senior nurse and a physiotherapist was of help to them. The study was designed with advice from an experienced clinical psychologist who then went on to carry out separate semi-structured interviews with both the patient and spouse or partner at home. The whole team were surprised by the main findings. Although it was well known that women are on average 10 years older than men when they suffer a heart attack, the social consequences had not been appreciated. Women patients attending the cardiac rehabilitation sessions were single or widowed and if they had worked, were retired. This was in contrast to men who usually had the support of their spouse or partner and were working prior to suffering their heart attack. Also most women had to take care of themselves following discharge from hospital whereas most men were looked after by their wife or partner. The age and social difference left the women feeling isolated and less able to engage in the rehabilitation group sessions. Many of the women said it was case of "all the boys together."

This study led to major changes in the way cardiac rehabilitation was delivered, ensuring that the program was more inclusive and would meet the needs of all heart attack patients.

EXPERIMENTAL RESEARCH

The word "experimental" immediately suggests images of laboratory studies but it can apply equally to healthcare research. Studies which involve exposing matched groups of patients to different treatment interventions is a form of experimental research. Usually one group of patients receive active treatment and their responses are compared to those of a second group who remain untreated (in the case of a drug trial, they receive a matching placebo tablet). Alternatively, and nowadays more often, a new treatment intervention will be compared to existing conventional treatment. A simple comparison study or trial involves random allocation to either the treatment or placebo arm, the allocation being known to both the patient and investigator (an open randomized clinical trial). Clearly, bias will be a problem and adopting a single-blind design, in which only the investigator knows what treatment the patient is receiving, minimizes this problem.

A double-blind approach is better still and the double-blind randomized controlled trial (RCT) design is the gold standard for assessing a new drug or comparing drug treatments. RCTs can be carried out using small or large groups of patients, depending the aim of the study. Outcome studies, for example, with endpoints such as the effects of treatment interventions on heart attack or stroke will require the recruitment of very large numbers of patients. By contrast, a study comparing the blood pressure-lowering effects of two drugs could be undertaken in one center. A small group size RCT may sometimes include a cross-over from one treatment to another with a wash-out period between the two arms. These are usually short-term studies with a treatment period of no more than 8–12 weeks with a short wash-out period of perhaps 2–4 weeks. The cross-over design can be useful in small group studies but treatment carry-over effects from one period to the next may occur. Appropriate statistical analysis will ensure that a carry-over has had no significant effect on the results.

Getting started in research

The majority of students find their first foray into research a daunting prospect and it is helpful to break down the development of a project into a series of steps.

All research starts with an idea. This may have occurred to you during clinical practice or may be one suggested by your supervisor. Either way, you should undertake a literature search before developing the idea in discussion with your supervisor. But most importantly, choose a topic which is of interest to you.

Frame a research question which is not too ambitious or broad based and is capable of achieving an answer in the time available for the project.

It is essential to search the literature and provide a relevant literature review. This is a time-consuming process and you need to employ systematic search criteria. It will help you to develop your research idea and provide the evidence to justify your study to the research ethics committee and introduce your study in a scientific and informative way. A critical review of the literature also will:

- give you a greater understanding of the topic you propose to research
- help you decide on the most appropriate research design
- ensure that your research question has not been answered by someone else.

Evaluating the literature is always challenging because you have to make a decision about relevance and whether the article you are reading is trustworthy. The best research papers appear in peer-reviewed journals such as *The Lancet*, *Pain*, *Manual Therapy*, etc. One can expect that these are reliable sources but nonetheless it is essential for you to make your critical of all these articles.

Important considerations include the following.

- Sample size (will the study have sufficient statistical power?).
- Recruitment of participants (are they representative of the population which you plan to study?).
- Research design (is it based on a systematic review of high-quality RCTs with meta-analysis or an expert's opinion?).
- Control of variables.
- Statistics (is the statistical analysis appropriate?).
- Follow-up (carry-over of effects).
- Age of study (is it too old to consider?).
- Did it answer the research question?
- Conflict of interest (do the results serve a deeper purpose?).

It is hoped that you will have now fully justified your study idea using the best available evidence. However, you should always check with your supervisor before moving on to develop a research protocol.

Developing a research protocol involves choosing appropriate methodology and ensuring adequate patient group sizes. Statistical advice is best sought at the project design stage, particularly where treatment comparisons are to be made. Many studies fail because patient group sizes are inadequate with the result that there is insufficient statistical power to demonstrate a treatment effect.

Seek a research ethics committee (REC) review and approval. A submission to the REC requires a copy of the research protocol, a patient information leaflet and consent form. All research involving patients can only proceed after the protocol has received approval from the REC. This applies to all projects, including the administration of patient questionnaires.

Clearly, developing a research idea into a full project together with obtaining approval from the local REC can take many months. Students need to start planning for their project well in advance to avoid delaying the start of their research. It is essential that students have regular contact with their supervisor during the whole process to ensure it all goes smoothly with no hitches.

SUMMARY OF RESEARCH PROJECT DEVELOPMENT

- Develop a research idea.
- Frame an appropriate question.
- Write a full research protocol with a patient information leaflet and consent form.
- Make an early submission for research ethics committee review.
- Once approval from the REC has been granted, then, and only then, can the research project get under way. Now the really exciting part of the whole project begins.

Good luck with your research project. You may surprise yourself and get hooked on research long term.

Real-life researchers

Each of the researchers mentioned in this section is an active research physiotherapist. They are either completely research/university based or find a mixture of research and clinical work.

Many newly qualified professionals decide quite quickly that they never want to think about research again – quite understandable considering that most health professional qualifying degrees end with a massive research dissertation! However, most realize that research is more than reading through reams of previous papers and literature reviews. It actually can contribute considerably to the way we work. For example, Nick Harland began working in a spinal unit and found himself using an outcome measure recommended by a consultant surgeon. "I was doing an MSc and had an interest in outcome measurement so took a look at the suggested tools and thought they were poor. I presented to various people including our surgeon and governance." Dr Harland had completed a form of research – a literature review. As such, Dr Harland's suggestion was accepted and the standard outcome measure was implemented – the Coping Strategies Questionnaire (CSQ). Dr Harland's ambition, however, drove him to consider further options in the interest of convenience and efficiency "Though I knew the CSQ was one of the best tools of its kind out there and had chosen it as such, its length and complex scoring irritated me so I independently undertook research, with data gained from my MSc dissertation that was an extensive longitudinal audit of our outcomes, and came up with a more valid, shorter and clinically useful version of the CSQ: the CSQ24. I published this with a little stats help in 2003. Since then the tool has had international uptake and so I started a PhD on the subject." Dr Harland's updated CSQ24 has been recognized as the coping tool of choice and recommended following independent research from the University of South Australia for the New Zealand government. Despite never having worked as a "researcher," Nick managed to identify a shortcoming in practice and implement change with startling results. He concludes: "It started with not wanting to be told what to do, then was followed by a clinical need for a better tool, and the rest is history."

Another drive for research in the clinical setting is the need to ensure that treatments are of the highest quality and the most effective. While the NHS is, of course, a setting for this, sports medicine is a particularly high-pressured environment for clinicians of all disciplines due to the unusual stresses placed upon the body of the patient. Craig Ranson is Chief Physiotherapist with UK Athletics and the former National Lead Physiotherapist with the England and Wales Cricket Board. Dr Ranson talks about his research achievement, "the highlight being the Grammer Award for the best 2006 basic science paper in European Spine Journal." Dr Ranson makes it clear that having an interest in research, and indeed being an active researcher, fosters vigilance in your clinical effectiveness. "I definitely believe that being a researcher has enhanced my clinical abilities, effectiveness and career progression in a variety of ways," he says.

He gives the following examples of the benefits of research in a clinical setting.

- Writing requires you to discover, understand and look critically at the literature on cutting-edge practice.
- In sport, being able to use injury surveillance statistics to identify problem injuries and prioritize injury prevention programs has made practice more effective (also evidenced by the stats).
- Investigating the relationships between quantifiable musculoskeletal risk factors and injury allows precise identification of, and interventions for, at-risk athletes.
- Being able to demonstrate to employers that the above can be used to develop strategic objectives and measures of effectiveness for physio departments has certainly helped my career progress.

Research as a primary job description is becoming more popular with new graduates too. As more challenging employment prospects loom and universities enhance the student's scientific understanding, recently qualified physiotherapy researchers are more numerous. One such researcher is Linzy Houchen who is based in Leicester. She graduated in 2006 and soon joined a cardiopulmonary specialist center as a principal investigator and is currently completing a PhD. Ms Houchen states her main fears regarding this step as:

- lack of research experience
- lack of support and isolation
- losing other skills
- questionable long-term career options.

However, Ms Houchen soon discovered that by making contact with colleagues, asking for help and engaging with the regulatory and governing body and clinical interest groups, these fears were soon quelled. She added that the benefits of researching are:

- pursuit of an area of interest and becoming an expert
- more negotiable study leave
- possibility of further qualifications – PhD, Doctor of Physiotherapy, etc.
- dedicated research time
- international travel and funded conference places.

May Nel is a cardiopulmonary physiotherapist in London who for many years believed that postgraduate education/research was "for the great ones, the gurus – never for me." Ms Nel found that her practice was becoming rather boring, to the extent that she became complacent, so she decided to undertake an MSc in advanced cardiopulmonary physiotherapy. "Since qualifying, I have had the opportunity to present a poster, abstract and an article. I am also a principal investigator for a Department of Health funded study." She adds, "My enthusiasm for research and knowledge has gained great impetus since completing the MSc and my team are reaping the benefits too." To conclude, Ms Nel makes the point that you don't have to be important or particularly clever to do research and that although it is hard work, it enriches your practice, making work a fulfilling and meaningful endeavor.

Further reading

Hicks, C., 2005. Research Methods for Clinical Therapists, fourth ed. Churchill Livingstone Elsevier, Edinburgh.
Porter, S., 2008. First Steps in Research. Churchill Livingstone Elsevier, Edinburgh.

The degree continues
Nick Southorn and Nick Clode

- Professional practice 144
- Evidence-based practice 145
- Portfolio development 147
- Reflection 154

The final stretch

Now that you are flying through the degree, some issues other than the human sciences and disease come to mind. Professional practice, research, evidence-based care, etc. all play a huge part in shaping you as a clinician. These will be emphasized by your course tutors and your clinical educators. Although it may seem boring right now, ultimately it will enhance your ability to provide exceptional care for your patients that is supported by best evidence. It is very much worth getting to grips with it all now rather than later.

As you are coming to the end of your studies, you should be considering an elective placement, if you haven't already done so. Not all universities offer an elective placement but I have included it here just in case.

Professional practice

Physiotherapists are primary care professionals. Being a medical professional involves (Koehn 1994):

- licensure to practice from the state
- autonomy over practice (i.e. you make your own mind up regarding treatment based upon your knowledge)
- belonging to a regulatory professional body which sets out strict rules of professional conduct and behavior
- having knowledge and skills not possessed by others (i.e. a defined scope of legal practice that can only be performed by that profession)
- a commitment to assist those in need.

Physiotherapy encompasses all these aspects in most of the world. One of the most important points is clinical autonomy: the legal right to assess, diagnose and treat patients according to your own knowledge and expertise. This comes with immense responsibility, making the physiotherapist accountable for their actions. In these times of litigation we must be mindful of what we do and say at all times. This brings in another factor of professionalism – belonging to a professional body that provides rules and regulations to adhere to and removes from the register those who fail to do so. These rules essentially provide you with the legal framework to work to; if you step outside it you are doing so *not* as a professional and as such will not benefit from support from your peers should action be brought against you. My advice is to visit the regulatory body relevant to you, and read and digest its rules of professional conduct, code of ethics, core standards, guide for professional conduct, etc. as they are so very important to you. Really – I'm not kidding!

You will notice in these professional regulations that you are about to have a big old pile of responsibility. But aren't they all just common sense? Well, effectively, yes! *You* know that you will respect the patient's confidentiality, be understanding and considerate, do no harm, act within your scope, etc. but how does the patient know that? What if they feel that you *didn't* respect their condition or inflicted harm?

Something that will become apparent during your years of study is the fact that physiotherapists seldom work alone. Recognition and respect for this fact are the first step to becoming a great clinician. Other team members will range from clinical professionals such as doctors, occupational therapists and psychologists through the social professionals such as social workers, addiction workers and hairdressers to the friends and carers of the patient. It goes without saying that each member of this multidisciplinary team, or MDT, is as important as the next.

The keystone of team work is communication. Inefficient or incorrect notes, messages, etc. *will* lead to a breakdown in effective care. All it takes is for one member not to complete the notes in a timely way or to forget to inform a team member of a change of routine and the whole thing falls flat. And who suffers? You guessed it – the patient.

Take note

Good note keeping is not only to provide adequate information for your colleagues. It is an essential part of professional practice. By recording everything, you are protecting yourself should any litigatory proceedings be taken against you and providing means for good continuity of care for the patient. You are also noting the objective markers – there is no point whatsoever taking measurements and then forgetting them all! Lastly, a good plan noted at the end of each session will direct you nicely when the patient returns to your clinic. Most clinicians (of all professions) find note taking laborious but by understanding the rationale and developing your own style, you will soon be writing perfect notes without breaking sweat.

Another barrier to cohesive working is poor knowledge of colleagues' expertise. I'm not saying you should attempt a full psychologic profile of the patient before referring to a psychologist but knowing what they will do will vastly decrease the number of embarrassingly inappropriate referrals made. A nice way to do this is to spend time with the professional. Make friends with them, talk to them, i.e. communicate!

You are likely to meet professionals who appear not to value the contribution of other team members; this is tricky! Maintain your integrity – they are the ones at fault as they clearly don't understand and respect other roles. The best way to defeat this kind of inappropriate behavior depends on who is affected. If it is just your feelings then swallow your pride and continue to provide top-notch care to your patient and stop caring about what other people think. If it is affecting patient care then speaking to a senior will help resolve any professionally related issues. Alternatively, more senior colleagues may advise that you speak directly to said ignoramus to resolve the issue. This is generally good advice but this must be done with the explicit support of your senior physiotherapist – don't try to "wing it" on your own!

Evidence-based practice

Evidence-based practice is the basis of modern healthcare. It is the delivery of treatment that is proven by high-quality research in both scientific laboratory and clinical settings. The days of unqualified claims of cure-alls are over for respectable professionals but unfortunately some types of treatment are still subscribed to by the general public despite significant scientific evidence that they are of no use. Leave these treatments to the charlatans out there and put your energy into physiotherapy.

Evidence-based practice is a big deal for physiotherapists. In the 1980s and 1990s the profession was rightly criticized for not providing proof that our techniques work; of course, we had empiric evidence, in that we observed improvements in our patients, but little in the way of published scientific research. Now, I am glad to say, more and more physiotherapists are making use of their scientific training and providing high-quality research. Some of the techniques have low-grade evidence and therefore are no longer used by conscientious professionals. However, the more we as a profession break down research barriers and develop our skills, scope and practice, the more we and our patients will benefit.

Sources of research are all over the place, just visit your library journal section and prepare to be bowled over! Now, as you are hard-working people who have already completed large amounts of scientific study, I don't need to tell you that you can't just take an article, read the abstract and conclusion and be happy that you are now up to date on that particular subject. You always need to search the databases and gather as much research on the topic as you can and extract the most relevant research before selecting the best study based upon a number of criteria using a standard appraisal tool and rank them by their quality. Usually a high-quality randomized controlled trial (RCT) or systematic review with meta-analysis of RCTs is considered the gold standard in research and case studies are simply used to generate a hypothesis rather than prove treatment efficacy. Alternatively you can see if someone has done it for you on the Cochrane database (a high-quality service providing reviews of past research). Thorough, objective and systematic searches are essential to produce nonbiased conclusions regarding treatment of a condition.

While you are at university it is advisable to get together with friends and form a journal group. The idea is that you pick a topic, let's say physiotherapy treatment of lateral epicondylitis. Then you all brainstorm for possible search terms such as "manual therapy," "lateral epicondylitis," "tennis elbow," "electrotherapy," "physical therapy," etc. and for databases to search such as Cochrane or Ovid. Then, between you, you share out the possible treatments. The idea is that you all go away and carry out the search as per the set criteria and gather the results. Once you have siphoned out the irrelevant stuff, you will be left with a few highly relevant and useful papers. With these, you write a synopsis and present back to your group with a conclusion as to whether or not that particular treatment is clinically worthwhile. By doing this, you are ensuring that you are always on the ball with current thinking and theories. Starting this at university will set you in the right direction for when you begin work and this type of behavior is expected from you.

Of course, you don't have to go to these lengths. Working on your own has real benefits in terms of you having control over what you learn. However, with research papers you will need to develop a way of making them accessible to you. Reading these things is a drag – scientific prose is purposefully dull and when you read two or three in a session, you may find that you haven't been paying attention for the last few pages. Highlighters and sticky notes are always useful! However, keep revisiting the conclusions you came to and see if you still remember why you would select a certain treatment for a specific patient – this is also part of clinical reasoning.

Portfolio development

N. Clode

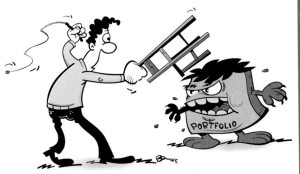

Fig. 13.1 Get your portfolio under control as soon as you can. The longer you leave it, the harder it gets.

What is a CPD portfolio?

It is pertinent to start off by first addressing what is meant by the term continuous professional development (CPD) and why it is so relevant to the physiotherapy profession. Physiotherapists have an obligation to their patients to ensure they are giving a high standard of care by using evidence-based practice in combination with learning from their ongoing professional experience. The field of research is continuously developing and evolving with new evidence constantly being produced. In order to stay abreast of these changes, an individual must maintain the practice of continual learning and career-long development. To ensure that learning undertaken is effective and relevant to an individual's role, it should be structured, recorded and evaluated. A system should also be in place to provide a vehicle through which future learning requirements are identified and where learning and its impact on practice can be evidenced. The CPD portfolio is the recommended tool for achieving these goals. The Chartered Society of Physiotherapy (CSP) refers to a portfolio as a "private collection of evidence that demonstrates learning and development as well as a tool for planning future learning" (CSP 2008, p4).

The questions which most physiotherapy students ask when starting the process of portfolio keeping are "What it should look like?", "What should I include in a portfolio?" and "How do I get started?". There are no strict rules as a portfolio is meant to be entirely individual to its owner. This can make it hard for tutors to articulate to students exactly what to do to start the process of portfolio keeping. The lack of boundaries or rules for keeping a CPD portfolio can sometimes cause students to become confused or neglect this important subject until after they finish their degree. Consequently, they may miss the experience of steering learning and taking responsibility for this important aspect of individual development from an early point in their degree. Some universities incorporate portfolio keeping into their undergraduate physiotherapy curriculum to familiarize their students with the process of portfolio keeping. However, a large number do not. This section has been written to help students understand the basics of portfolio keeping and get started with a practical approach to keeping a CPD portfolio. For a more comprehensive guide to portfolio keeping, have a look at the resources at the end of the chapter.

Why do I need to keep a CPD portfolio?

The professional body for physiotherapy, the CSP, expects that its members continually learn throughout their careers in order to maintain competence as part of their professional code of conduct. Whilst the CSP expects its members use a CPD portfolio, until recently there has not been a structured process that regulates whether physiotherapists are undertaking CPD practices. Due to the modernization of the health service and the government's push towards raising standards of patient care, the regulatory body for allied health professionals (including physiotherapists), the Health Professions Council (HPC), has started auditing whether their registrants are undertaking and maintaining up-to-date records of CPD activities. All physiotherapists in the United Kingdom legally have to be registered with the HPC to practice physiotherapy in any setting. When registering and re-registering with the HPC, physiotherapists must sign a legal document stating that they meet the HPC standards for CPD, including the maintenance of an up-to-date record of CPD activities. From April 2010, every 2 years, a random sample of 2.5% of the physiotherapy profession will be asked to submit evidence to demonstrate that they meet the CPD standards. This does not mean an individual has to submit their entire CPD portfolio, but they must provide written evidence of ongoing learning and how this has contributed to improvements in practice. Registrants are expected to draw parts out of their CPD portfolio to help complete what the HPC calls a CPD profile.

Physiotherapy students do not have to be registered with the HPC and therefore do not have any auditing process to go through apart from that which their universities require. It is pertinent, however, to ensure that you are prepared for the professional obligation of self-directing, maintaining and evidencing learning practices by becoming familiar with keeping a CPD portfolio throughout your time as a student.

What does a portfolio look like?

Traditionally most physiotherapists have used a large A4 ring binder, broken down into sections containing plastic wallets which can be used to simply insert and withdraw relevant papers, certificates, reflections, etc. However, electronic portfolios are now gaining popularity which has prompted the CSP to release their own web-based version called PebblePad. There are advantages and disadvantages to both electronic and paper-based systems and it is up to you which one you use. Most physiotherapy students are comfortable with using information technology so it is assumed the majority will prefer using the online version. The merits of the online and paper-based portfolio systems will be discussed below.

What should it contain?

The simple answer to this question is anything that evidences your professional or personal development. Basic things that you can include with little or no extra work are certificates of qualifications, training courses, events attended, past achievements and evidence from appraisals that are undertaken on clinical placements or essay reports/feedback. You will spend the latter part of your physiotherapy degree writing critical appraisals of research papers or current treatment techniques, all of which make valuable entries to your portfolio. After clinical placements you will likely be asked to reflect and write reports on patient cases or significant incidents which demonstrate what you learned and how your practice changed after the event; these make great evidence of learning and its impact on practice. Other standard material that may be incorporated into a CPD portfolio are peer reviews that you perform with your student colleagues, written comments from patients on placements or learning style questionnaires that can be used to identify the best way for you to learn. Ideas for suitable CPD material have been summarized in the box on page 153.

These recommendations are simply suggestions but will help you to make a start and add a bit of bulk to your portfolio, which in my experience is the most intimidating part of portfolio keeping! If you've just started your degree and do not have much evidence so far, do not worry. Just follow the steps included at the end of the chapter to set up a CPD portfolio and add your current academic certificates or relevant awards/certification of attendance, collecting the rest of the material as you continue throughout your degree.

The final important point is that your portfolio is supposed to be an *up-to-date* record of learning, so try to include material that is not more than 2 years old. This means you will have to allocate time every so often to review the contents of your portfolio and remove outdated material.

> TIP: If using a paper-based portfolio system, buy a spare file to use as a "reference file" to keep all the material you take out of your portfolio as it becomes outdated.

Portfolio keeping – what you need to know

The most important thing is to start the process of portfolio keeping and begin to understand the relevance of a portfolio as a tool for learning and development. It is easy enough to buy a folder and store certificates, reports, reflections and other pieces of university work to evidence CPD. The more challenging part of portfolio keeping is how you use it as a tool for personal/professional development. To this end, you should use the material stored in a portfolio to assist you in identifying learning requirements, assessing the impact of learning on your practice and evidence your ongoing development. The CSP provides a useful model to assist with the planned learning process. This can be applied to any individual/situation and contains the underpinning structure for planned learning.

Figure 13.2 shows the CSP's planned learning process model (CSP 2001) along.

The CSP also provides pro formas which assist with the CPD process and can be accessed by CSP members. These are forms containing questions that

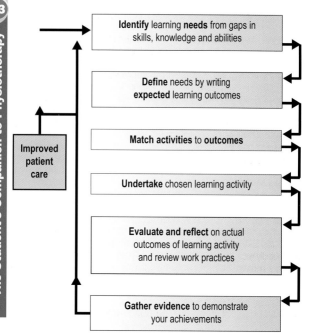

are simple to fill in and assist the user with planning learning, reflecting and assessing expertise, amongst other areas. These are useful to get an idea of what is expected when undertaking an entry into a CPD portfolio and can be downloaded from the CSP's online portfolio system (http://eportfolio.csp.org.uk/) or via the CSP's portfolio of learning CD-ROM. These are only templates and are open to modification. You may also want to make your own, but the pro formas may save you time and help give you direction when reflecting upon or planning learning. Other useful CPD pro formas can be obtained from hospitals whilst on clinical placements, so it's worth asking what forms your fellow clinicians use to assist their CPD and take a blank photocopy of any you see that you feel might be valuable.

The other important fact of which to be aware is that not all learning is planned and structured. Useful learning experiences arise incidentally every day from discussions with peers and tutors or from treating patients on placements. Incidental or informal learning experiences are just as valid as the formal, structured learning and can be recorded and reflected upon to ensure that learning is evidenced and to assess how it has impacted upon practice. This does not require you to write lengthy reflective essays which are commonly completed as part of an academic course, but a few lines or bullet points describing what happened, what you learned and how this will impact on your future practice would be sufficient to provide an entry in your CPD portfolio. If possible, a later piece of evidence could then be included to show how this learning has been integrated into your practice. I think one of the main things that deters students from undertaking CPD practices separate to their degree is the perception that portfolio keeping is a lengthy process, when this doesn't have to be the case.

It is important to note that when considering what evidence to include or what chosen learning activity is most appropriate, no single CPD activity is superior and it will depend on a variety of factors such as your learning style, previous methods of learning used, learning outcomes, time and resources which dictate what particular learning medium is selected for a given activity. The CSP recommends attempting to include evidence from a variety of different activities (CSP 2005).

HINT: You could look at the summary of methods of learning in the box on page 000 and try to include evidence from five different sources within your portfolio.

There is an additional factor to take into account with regard to portfolio keeping. When attending job interviews for newly qualified positions, physiotherapy employers often ask applicants to bring their CPD portfolio. Not all employers make this request as a portfolio is meant to be your individual record of learning and you would be within your rights to refuse. However, as you will undoubtedly want to come across as open and forthcoming, I personally feel that having a portfolio that is appropriately organized and which you are willing to share is important when hunting for that first job.

Online versus paper-based portfolio systems

ONLINE PORTFOLIO KEEPING

Advantages of the electronic portfolio system is that it avoids the need to store large volumes of paper and the portfolio can be accessed anywhere that has a computer with internet access. Using the online system, you do not need to review the portfolio as regularly as the paper-based system to remove outdated work, as there is a large online storage capacity. This can be a relatively time-consuming task when using a paper-based portfolio system. When you do need to filter outdated information from PebblePad, it can be simply saved and stored on a pen drive, disk or hard drive.

The online portfolio can be used to create and store a curriculum vitae and has simple questionnaires to complete which can help you identify areas for personal and professional development. Electronic information can be uploaded from computer hard drives, disks, pen storage devices or the internet quickly and easily onto the portfolio, which means you do not need to print documents out and amendments can be made simply. You can also allow others access to your site to view parts of your portfolio for comment or peer review. The help facility is very clear and easy to use which is handy when you're a novice and I would recommend taking some time to visit this initially to view the system's capabilities. However, you will need audio speakers to get the full benefit.

Drawbacks with using the online portfolio are similar to anything IT based. That is, you will need regular access to a computer with an internet connection. Further, you will need certain downloadable software and good web browser speed. It is assumed that not all students will have a computer available at home which could be problematic if you wanted to update your portfolio in the evening after you get home from university. The system is very comprehensive so it can take a significant period of time to become familiar with how to use it, which may make portfolio keeping slower initially than compiling a paper-based portfolio. Many paper documents such as academic certificates, course handouts, copies of patients' notes, reports and appraisals will have to be scanned into a computer or kept separately in a file, which may be inconvenient if a scanner is not readily available.

PAPER-BASED PORTFOLIOS

The advantages of using paper-based portfolios are that certificates, essays, reflections, etc. can be simply inserted into the file. Paper-based systems are quick to set up and have the flexibility for the individual to use artistic license to create their own sections and display material however they like. Most importantly, they can be shown to future employers as evidence of commitment to CPD.

If you choose to establish a paper-based portfolio you could use a ring binder, box file, professional portfolio (obtainable from a stationery shop) or anything that can be used to segment and store information. As mentioned earlier, there are no hard-and-fast rules on what a portfolio should look like and strictly speaking, you are not obliged to show it to anyone else (only extracts out of the portfolio to use as evidence of CPD for HPC re-registration requirements). However, as most people take their portfolios to job interviews (this is sometimes stated as a prerequisite for interviews), it is worth remembering that you may be judged on its appearance. A well-presented, organized portfolio may be easier for you to manage and will demonstrate to employers that you are committed to CPD.

Overall, I think the best bet is to start off using the electronic system to save and store all your computer-based assignments, reflections, professional communications, etc. but to create a paper-based system in tandem to keep paper copies of certifications, essay reports that you haven't scanned into a computer, etc.

Steps in setting up a CPD portfolio

- Sign in to the CSP online portfolio via the icon on the homepage of the CSP website: www.csp.org.uk/. Note: You have to be a CSP member to use the online portfolio and have a username and password. If you have forgotten this information, contact the CSP enquiries handling unit on 0207 314 7890 or email them at www.enquiries@csp.org.uk/.

- Browse through the help facility to familiarize yourself with the facilities available within the online system.

And/or:

- buy a large A4 ring binder or equivalent
- purchase 100+ plastic wallets and 10 file dividers
- decide on section titles (see box below), insert file dividers and labels, create an index page
- insert relevant documents.

Ideas for sections in a paper-based portfolio

- **Personal information** Personal statement, CV
- **Learning requirements** Learning needs analysis
- **Learning objectives** Developmental objectives
- **Certifications** Academic certificates, awards
- **Events attended** Study days, CSP Congress
- **Reflections** Reflective essays
- **Critical appraisal** Appraisal of research studies
- **Professional practice** Placement grades, feedback
- **Other** Voluntary, work experience

This is a limited list and should be adapted to suit the individual portfolio.

HINT: As a student you aren't expected to do a large amount of extracurricular work to add to your portfolio as your learning is somewhat directed by the higher education institution and it is taken for granted that you will be progressing knowledge and skills throughout your physiotherapy degree. Make sure you start putting relevant pieces of university work into a portfolio as early as possible so that you won't have to hunt for old pieces of work, clinical reports, reflections from previous years that you put down somewhere and which have disappeared into your room, never to be seen again!.

Ideas for material that can be included within a CPD portfolio

- Curriculum vitae
- Academic certificates
- Certification of achievements, e.g. voluntary work, awards, etc.
- Feedback from assignments
- Personal tutor meetings, feedback
- Clinical supervisors' comments
- Observation placements, reflections
- Discussions with colleagues, tutors, clinicians relating to professional issues
- Copies of in-service training presentations
- Critical appraisal of journal articles
- Reflections, reflective essays
- Peer reviews
- Learning objectives
- Learning styles questionnaire
- Self-audits (e.g. SWOT analysis)
- Literature reviews
- Letters of praise from service users!

Finally

As a physiotherapy student, your main focus should be on establishing a basic portfolio and developing an understanding of how to manage and structure your individual learning. Establishing and maintaining a CPD portfolio can seem like a burden alongside your academic studies and may not feel like a priority. However, following the steps within this chapter can allow you to minimize the work you need to do and completing small bits often can save a lot of time in the long run. During my own training, it wasn't until I realized I wouldn't get all the knowledge I needed during my studies to practice competently as a band 5 physiotherapist that I started to invest more of my time in "learning how to learn"!

Reflection

Reflection … you either know about it or you don't: either way, the chances are that you are a reflective person anyway. Put rather simply, reflection is analyzing our performance with a view to improving on it the next time, i.e. learning from our mistakes! The aim is to improve service delivery, skills, team work, etc. and eventually increase your feeling of accomplishment. As a normal member of society, I guess that is all you need to know – but you are no longer a normal member of society, you are a health professional (well, nearly). Reflecting as a professional requires time and effort in order to do it properly; more importantly, it requires a pen and paper or keyboard and screen. It should serve as a platform from which you can begin your journey of improvement and as a reminder of how far you have come. Before I go on, it is worth remembering that you don't only have to reflect upon events which you feel went badly – you can reflect on things that you did well in order to analyze *what* you did so well, *why* you did so well and *how* you can do so again.

Adequate reflection involves a good deal of description. You must develop the skill of describing an event in a completely objective and independent way (i.e. a description is literally "what happened" with no other information needed). This is essential for you to set the scene and can be done in a story format, bullet point format, etc.; you may want to list the people who were present at the time and so on. This helps you to process the series of events logically; perhaps when you think about an event in such detail something will become apparent that you may not have remembered previously. That is a fundamental part of reflection: analysis and reanalysis to foster a more detailed understanding.

You will need to identify the significance of the event; for example, if it is a presentation you gave to your peers then it is hugely significant as it may alter how people think of you; presentations are something that you may be expected to do quite a lot in the future and therefore you need to be confident that you can do it well. Whatever the event and its significance, try to widen it to a broader context as well; can you apply what you have learned in other situations?

Describe how you felt at the time, a couple of days later once you had thought about it for a while and now, as you write the reflective piece. Consider how your changes in attitude to what happened may reflect upon how significant the event *really* was to you.

You will want to consider the thoughts and feelings of other people – the patient, colleagues, your employer, etc.– even if they weren't there at the time. How would they feel about the event? You may even wish to talk to these people to gather actual input rather than inferred input.

You can reflect on how the incident has affected you since, perhaps even how you reflected upon it! How did it make you feel to relive the event? You can dig deeper and deeper into reflective writing and ultimately you will come to a set of conclusions.

What will you do next time? Do you need to go away and learn about something? Did this event open your eyes to a weakness you didn't know you had? If so, why? The great thing about this is that you are the architect of your own learning and improvement. You have control and you can do something about it. Now go make some targets to meet relating to the reflection.

There are many "reflective tools" out there, too many to mention. Make yourself aware of them and if you happen to see one you like, perhaps you can use it. Many students prefer to look at these prescriptive tools simply for ideas and use the bits of each that suit them. You lecturers will guide you on what to look out for.

References

Chartered Society of Physiotherapy, 2001. CPD6 Developing a Portfolio: A Guide for CSP Members. Chartered Society of Physiotherapy, London.

Chartered Society of Physiotherapy, 2005. CPD30 The CPD process. Chartered Society of Physiotherapy, London.

Chartered Society of Physiotherapy, 2008. PD010 Keeping a Portfolio: Getting Started. Chartered Society of Physiotherapy, London.

Koehn, D., 1994. The Ground of Professional Ethics. Routledge, London.

Further reading

Health Professions Council, 2006. Continuing Professional Development and Your Registration. Health Professions Council, London.

14

You think it's all over ...
Nick Southorn and Nick Clode

- Results   158
- What to do with your textbooks   159
- Opportunities for the graduate   159
- Looking for jobs in the UK   160
- Interviews   162
- Conclusion   170

The final stretch

It is now! So, exams are over and it's time to consider what is immediately important: your friends. You have all been through so much lately and soon you will see them less and less. Therefore, it's time to relax, party and generally enjoy the time between finishing the last exam and graduating. Easy to say, eh? I know, but here are a few short bits of parting advice that may help. I have purposefully left this chapter short because you should be spending this time with your future colleagues, remembering the good old days from when you thought you'd trip up in the lecture theater on day one to the many bodily fluids you encountered on placements!

Results

Awaiting the results in your final year is probably the most nerve-racking thing you have done in a while; yes; more nerve racking than waiting to hear if you have been accepted in to physio school or not! Some universities are very good and you have your results (or at least an indication as to whether or not you have passed) within a day or two. Some universities, however, take their sweet time over it! It's just one of those things and there is nothing you can do except sit back and party with your friends who you are going miss dearly in a few weeks' time.

However, I think you should consider this question: would the tutors *really* let a poorly performing student get this far unnoticed? The answer is No! If your tutor has not had to haul you in and give you a reality check in the last 3 or 4 years, the chances are you are going to pass. This is of course easy for me to say now I've passed … I was a nightmare waiting for my results (my university was in the latter category in taking its time over presenting results). It's never as bad as you convince yourself it's going to be. A close friend of mine was so convinced that he had failed, he rang his parents to stop them flying from Canada to see him graduate … he got a first class honors degree!

If you genuinely think that you may have messed up in an exam then don't panic – just go straight to your tutor who will help you in any way they can.

The majority of UK pre-registration courses are Bachelor of Science honors degrees, BSc (Hons), or a variant of that (such as Bachelor of Health Sciences). Honors graduates are awarded classes of degree – first, second (two divisions: upper and lower), and third. You can also graduate from your degree without honors if you fall below the third class banding or fail the research component of your degree (specific to physiotherapy).

Those who have completed a Master of Science level pre-registration degree, i.e. those who have a previous biologic science degree, will gain a pass, merit or distinction although not all universities offer a merit. However, you guys will already have been through all of this and will be taking it easy right now!

For those universities which offer doctoral level pre-registration courses, the student will earn either a pass or a fail (sometimes a distinction is offered). Doctor of Physiotherapy degrees in the UK are postgraduate qualifications only.

Does any of this matter? Well, that depends on what you wish to do with your qualification. If you intend to become a university academic and research is your future then your previous academic performance may be considered to continue further postgraduate study such as Masters or PhD, DPhysio, etc. But if you just want to be a physio then largely, the answer is "no." Being good at exams does *not* make you a good clinician and employers appreciate this.

Do not be fooled into thinking that as a graduate and qualified physiotherapist, you are expected to know much about treating patients! Now is where all the learning really starts.

So, basic advice about your result and banding … worry not, it's not as big a deal as you might think. NB: do not think that this is an excuse to bunk off and scrape a pass because this attitude becomes immediately apparent to interviewers and the one thing that they *do* want is a hard worker who gives it all.

What to do with your textbooks

You will have accumulated quite a library of books over the last few years unless you have lived in the library or borrowed endlessly! It may be tempting to sell your books to more junior students or on a popular net-based auction – people do so because recent graduates of any subject are usually in massive debt, don't have the room to store books and think that as they are undergraduate books, they are surplus to requirements.

Well, I can tell you that graduating from physio school does not mean you know everything there is to know about physiotherapy. During your first 2 years of practice you will be referring to those books more often than you did as a student. Believe me, selling or binning your books and notes is a sure set-up for disaster.

Some of your tutors may still have their undergraduate textbooks; this is because even they do not presume to know it all to the extent that they can discard their textbooks. Plus there is a certain nostalgic value to your university textbooks. They hold a very powerful link to times past and every page has more than just information – it is a page of history and of memories. So in 20 years' time, with fond thoughts of your time at university, you may turn to these tattered old pages and cast your mind back to the fun you are having now.

Opportunities for the graduate

You are a qualified physiotherapist and therefore have many skills. I have already discussed the opportunities in Chapter 1 but I feel that now you have finished, it is time to consider your options in more detail.

Had enough of physiotherapy but don't want to start at the beginning?

It is true that not all graduates see the traditional "first post" as being their goal. Many newly qualified physiotherapists consider their degree more in terms of a coming of academia rather than a vocation, just like any other degree. The point I am making is that you are in no way tied to being a physiotherapist just because you are trained as such. A look in your local or national high-quality newspaper will soon reveal many opportunities for "a graduate." Being "a graduate" opens doors into a world of business and professional status that relies more on your ability to learn, research, adapt, solve problems and work in a team. The difference is, as a physiotherapy graduate you have these traits drilled into you!

Problem solving is what you do; by researching, adapting to best practice and team work, you make your patient better. If your university has adopted the so-called "problem-based learning" model then you are there already! You may not have appreciated it at the time but by saying "go and find out," your lecturer has been teaching you one of the most important lessons of all: how to independently get the answer. Don't be afraid to approach nontraditional settings because you are a physiotherapy graduate: it is not a prison sentence.

Options for the physiotherapist include the following.

- *Further study* – other taught postgraduate courses will supplement your physiotherapy degree and enhance your specialist knowledge. However, they may be costly and require you to complete junior rotations beforehand. In addition, while you are not practicing as a physiotherapist you will "deskill" which is why part-time courses are popular amongst clinicians.

- *Research* – this may be clinical as part of your job or 100% university based as part of a higher qualification such as a PhD. There is massive demand for this in physiotherapy and once you get into it, research is fun!

- *Junior posts (internship)* – junior physiotherapy posts allow you to consolidate and further expand on knowledge attained whilst at university and develop your clinical skills. This is the preferred route and rightly so – it gives you a chance to rotate around the specialist areas and develop a real-life interest based on experience. In addition, you can fill in the gaps of your knowledge.

- *Independent practitioner* – this is probably the least advisable route to take straight from university. Most individuals after graduating do not have the skills to provide an adequate service or compete in the business world against more experienced practitioners. However, there are some private organisations that offer trainee posts including on the job training and develop that might be suitable for some graduates. These are generally few and far between.

- *Industry* – e.g. medical rep. Completely nonclinical really unless you become a "clinical advisor" which would be a surprising appointment for someone with no experience. However, your expert knowledge of the human body and your ability to retain and use complex information will ensure that if you do opt for this type of work, you will do well.

- Veterinary physiotherapy – not many people realize that animals need rehab too! Postgraduate study is recommended and very much available.

There are many more routes to take – someone is always willing to employ an eager physiotherapist! If you see yourself heading in a "nontraditional" direction the best thing to do is contact a physio who did the same thing. I am certain they will be glad to advise you.

Looking for jobs in the UK

N. Clode

This chapter is mainly aimed at UK job seekers. It includes the main websites and strategies for job hunting. Although this is aimed at UK job seekers it is worth reading wherever you wish to work as your representative organization may offer similar services.

Websites

WWW.JOBS.NHS.UK

This should be your first stop when looking for a band 5 NHS job. You can get emails delivered directly to your email account detailing job descriptions and personal specifications for band 5 posts across England. Ensure you register with NHS Jobs before you qualify so you can get an idea of how regularly posts are advertised and determine whether you meet most of the criteria within the person specifications. This could help highlight any shortcomings in your skill-set or identify areas in which to improve your curriculum vitae to increase your chances of being short-listed for jobs. NB: It is worth noting that due to the volume of applicants looking on NHS Jobs, adverts have usually closed by the time the email notification has been sent to your individual email account. Therefore it is a good idea to check the NHS website by performing manual searches as frequently as possible (i.e. every day or two) to ensure you don't miss out.

WWW.JOBESCALATOR.COM/

This is the CSP's vacancy website and contains a broad range of work opportunities. Many of the opportunities advertised via this site tend to be international or work within private practice. It is definitely worth checking for newly qualified vacancies or opportunities. To take advantage of this you must be a member of the CSP and have registered with the CSP website: www.csp.org.uk.

WWW.HEALTHJOBSUK.COM/JOBS

This website advertises UK-based jobs at various bands. A large number of jobs on this website are advertised for NHS organizations and many include working for recruitment agencies. Basic grades jobs are limited on this website, though it is worth the occasional check because they do come up.

WWW.PHYSIOBOB.COM/

This website offers hundreds of jobs from around the UK and internationally. Jobs are mainly for private practice, recruitment agencies and independent healthcare providers. Given the nature of the jobs, most are band 6 and above but opportunities for newly qualified physiotherapists do appear on this website so it is definitely worth a regular review.

WWW.JOBS.SCOT.NHS.UK/JOBS/INDEX.CFM

This is the website to check if you intend on working in Scotland. Scottish NHS jobs are advertised exclusively on this website and will not be found on the main NHS Jobs website.

WWW.N-I.NHS.UK

This website provides a link to a number of different websites that can be used to discover physiotherapy vacancies in Northern Ireland. Whilst there is not an abundance of physiotherapy jobs, if you are interested in working in Northern Ireland this should be bookmarked as a "favorite" on your web-server.

PRIVATE ORGANISATIONS

With an ever increasing number of newly qualified physiotherapists finding employment opportunities in the private sector, it is pertinent to check the websites of private organizations websites. One of the best known private healthcare providers that has recently taken on a number of physiotherapy graduates is BUPA. It may also be pertinent to check your yellow pages for local organisations that may employ graduate Physiotherapists. An example of these are new CATS centres (clinical assessment and treatment centres) which are now performing a lot of elective orthopaedic operations and are in need of graduate Physiotherapists.

Recruitment agencies

There are a number of recruitment agencies that offer employment opportunities for physiotherapists. Agencies that accept new graduates include:

- Pulse: www.pulsejobs.com/uk/
- www.justphysio.co.uk

The websites included in this section provide a solid foundation from which you should find suitable vacancies for which to apply. It is important to note that the list is not exhaustive. If there is a particular organization within which you would like to work, it would be worthwhile making contact with the organization directly. That way you will get inside information about when and where job adverts are likely to be coming out. Consider emailing or posting a copy of your CV to these places and request they keep it on file and notify you of any suitable vacancies. Not all organizations will keep CVs but some will so it's definitely worth a try.

Interviews

N. Clode

So, you have just received a letter through the post (or an email) inviting you for a physiotherapy job interview. Congratulations! A big question I know you'll be asking is "How do I make sure I perform well at interview?" Well, like anything else in life, you will need thorough preparation and rehearsal. It is essential you allocate as much time as possible in your busy schedule for interview planning and practice. Don't sell yourself short here; you've worked hard for 3 years to get to this point and you don't want to risk not doing yourself justice at the interview. Most of your nonurgent commitments will have to be put to one side, that's how crucial thorough preparation is.

The main reason for having an interview is for the employer to ascertain whether an individual is suitable for a specific post within their organization. Feedback I've attained from physiotherapy managers suggests that there are three main factors they take into account when evaluating the suitability of a candidate.

- How well will this individual fit in with the team?

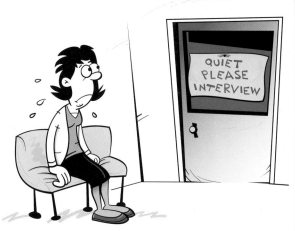

Fig. 14.1 Try not to be nervous – they are not there to make it hard for you. They must like you already otherwise you wouldn't be there in the first place!

- Can they do the job (knowledge, competence, safety, experience)?
- Will they do the job (motivation, commitment, enthusiasm, loyalty)?

It is up to you to show the interviewers that you're personable, a good team worker and will fit into whichever organization you are applying to, not always an easy task when you're nervous and feeling under pressure. To demonstrate competence, a number of methods can be employed, e.g. qualifications, grades at university, previous or current work experience, extracurricular/voluntary experience, references, reflections or awards within your CPD portfolio. Employers will also be interested in your personal qualities. You will need to show you're enthusiastic and that you have a specific interest in working for the particular organization. This can be achieved by showing that you've researched the organization so find out about local trust initiatives if applying to a hospital, or types of treatments offered if it's an independent practice. It is also worth having prepared examples of any accomplishments or experiences which show you are dynamic and interesting. This can include both physiotherapy-related and nonphysiotherapy-related achievements (charity/voluntary work, sporting activities, interests, representative roles) so get your thinking cap on!

Interview format

Recruitment procedures vary markedly between organizations and while most people have a preconception of what happens at an interview, experiences of graduates across the country have revealed that it is not always possible to know what you might be faced with on the day. The range of different formats which I and my peers have experienced include presentations in front of a board of interviewers, group interviews where 6–10 people are instructed to discuss a set topic amongst the group (e.g. how physiotherapists can contribute to the 18-week wait target), practical role plays where you are observed treating a dummy patient and written examinations including both short essays and multiple choice questions. Within an interview, the only thing you can guarantee is that there will be some form of oral component, where you will be asked questions face to face by your potential employers. As such, this chapter will in the main concentrate on preparing you for what is a "typical" 30-minute oral interview.

The majority of organizations commonly use 2–3 interviewers, though some candidates I've known have been unlucky enough to have up to six individuals making up the interview panel. These usually consist of physiotherapy managers, clinicians, ward managers, HR personnel, nonphysiotherapists (e.g. nurses) or in some inventive trusts even use service users (i.e. patients!). Interviews usually take place in the physiotherapy department at the trust or organizations main site, though they may occur in tertiary centers or within the human resources department so this is something you will need to find out as part of your preparation for the big day. I don't need to tell you that rushing around to find the interview site or underestimating traffic on the interview day isn't going to do your nerves any good!.

Preparation

In order to prepare adequately for an interview, you will need to know the kind of questions you will be asked and how to prepare so you are in the best position to answer these questions. A list of practice questions that have been asked of myself and other physiotherapy colleagues at interview can be found in the box below. Remember, every question has a purpose so analyze these questions carefully and consider the attributes for which the interviewer may be looking. Organizations may use standard interview questions or make the questions up themselves. That means you can never be sure what you're going to be asked. There is some preparation that should be done individually and some preparation for which you will need the help of other people.

Typical interview questions

- Tell us about yourself.
- Why did you choose a career in physiotherapy?
- What are your strengths and weaknesses in relation to physiotherapy?
- Tell us about your dissertation.
- How did you find your clinical placements?
- What do you feel is a band 5 physiotherapist's role in Clinical Governance?
- What is the Knowledge and Skills Framework?
- How would you prioritize treatment in a busy ward?
- Who is the most important person in a team?
- How would your friends describe you?
- Why would you like to work for the trust/organization?
- What has been your greatest achievement in the last year?
- What priority would you give to paperwork in a busy ward?

Interviewers need to be assured that a candidate has a sound theoretical knowledge of physiotherapy. Some will accept your physiotherapy degree as proof of your knowledge and competence, while a large majority will wish to test this at interview. This means you will more than likely benefit from some textbook swatting to ensure you are up to scratch for any clinical questions. The areas which you should study will depend specifically on the job for which you have applied. For example, if you are going for a junior rotational post, ensure you can answer questions in the "core" areas of musculoskeletal, respiratory, neurologic and orthopedic specialties. Alternatively, if you are applying for a job in a private practice you will need to ensure you are red hot at carry-out musculoskeletal assessments and treatments. Particular areas to focus on when preparing for generic clinical interview questions are assessment techniques, treatments and contraindications. It is common to be asked questions in the form of clinical scenarios. This helps determine not only your overall knowledge, but also your applied knowledge and common sense. Examples of specific clinical questions you might be asked are listed in the box below.

Clinical questions

- You are asked to see a 38-year-old female with pain in her cervical spine and anesthesia in her left hand. What are the possible pathologies related to these symptoms?

- What are the contraindications against using intermittent positive pressure breathing machines to treat atelectasis?

- You are working as a junior in a neurologic specialty, mobilizing a patient to the gym for treatment when they suddenly collapse. What do you do?

- What are the signs and symptoms of OA knee?

- Would you ever consider quality of movement over function with a post-stroke patient?

Another area which an applicant should study in order to prepare for an interview is organizational knowledge. As most readers of this text will probably be applying for jobs in the NHS, I will center discussion around this organization, but the principles mentioned could be applied to any other private or charitable organization.

An individual applying for a job within the NHS should be familiar with the frameworks and legislation which direct working practices within the NHS. At the time of writing, the main frameworks of note are Clinical Governance, Agenda for Change and the Knowledge and Skills Framework. There will also be current NHS targets which are usually driven by government White Papers and are frequently changing. These can be found by a simple search on the Department of Health website or just keeping a watchful eye on the national news. Study these areas until you have a sound understanding of the drivers and rationale behind each framework, then try to think of how this might impact upon the job for which you are applying. It may be beneficial to try to prepare examples.

Example: As a band 5 physiotherapist I can meet the standards dictated by Clinical Governance by:

1. ensuring confidentiality by appropriately securing paperwork in a safe place, not leaving patients' notes out on a desk and anonymizing patients' names when discussing patient cases with colleagues or seniors

2. considering infection control within my job, adopting the trust's local hand-washing procedures and patient protection protocols

3. ensuring equality and diversity legislation by respecting the rights and wishes of all individuals irrelevant of race, sex, age, ethnicity or social class. This may include treating certain ethnic patients fully clothed when undertaking MSK assessments or ensuring I am sensitive to body image issues when treating members of the opposite sex.

A decent practical tip I once got from one of my physiotherapy tutors was to buy an A4 file, place inside an abundance of plastic wallets and call this my "job file." This can be used to collate all the information you need to retain with regard to job applications. Included will be job descriptions, person specifications, tips on CV writing, interview questions or examples of other people's personal statements. This can be started as early as the second year of university and be used to record those very important contact details of physiotherapy professionals you meet whilst on clinical placement. It is also wise to store information about the trusts in which you have your placements, as these might be places where you attend interviews in the future. The file will help you organize your job hunting endeavors and ensure you have any information you need to hand. Whether you do this or not, *always* make sure to keep a copy of the personal specification for every job for which you send an application as this will be used to underpin any assessment you go through at interview.

Pick through the person specification of the job for which you are applying and draw out the main skills and attributes required by the post (it may help to underline key words). Then try to think of examples from your clinical placements or any previous work experience where you have demonstrated these attributes. This way you won't feel pressured to think on the spot in interviews. An appropriately performed interview should be structured to ascertain which individuals are most suited to the person specification for the particular post and by focusing your preparation around the personal specification, you can feel confident that you've covered a large part of the interview already!

You can also use the person specification or job description to generate interview questions yourself. You can use these to think of how you can demonstrate that you are the ideal applicant for their organization. Also if there's anything else you've done that might favorably impact on your application, think of how you might be able to bring this into the conversation (e.g. if you won an award, represented a group of people, did some related voluntary work). It is perfectly acceptable to attempt to exert some control over the interview, as long as you ensure that you suitably answer the question.

The last thing I would highly recommend is that you take the time and effort to go into the trust and ask the person who will be carrying out the interview a few pertinent questions. This may not be feasible in every case but will achieve three aims.

- It will ensure that there are no nasty surprises on interview day with regard to interview format, length and location.

- It demonstrates to the interviewer that you are keen, enthusiastic and proactive. They will no doubt remember this on the interview day.

- It will help you relax on the interview day as you will see a familiar face and surroundings and will have already had a chance to build some rapport with the interviewer.

While it may not always be possible to visit the organization in person, you can always pick up the telephone and ask to speak to one of the individuals performing the interview. You would be amazed how few candidates take the time to do this.

WORKING WITH OTHERS

While a large amount of preparation can be done independently, it is important to gain some experience talking in front of another person and preferentially a group of people. This can be anyone, ranging from family members (mum, dad, cousins, grandma) to complete strangers. The person doing the interviewing doesn't have to know about physiotherapy, but it is helpful to attempt to create as much of a formal atmosphere as possible. This will give you the greatest preparation for the interview day. Obviously if the person doing the interview is a physiotherapist then that may be better, as they will be able to provide feedback regarding the quality of clinical or NHS-related answers and suggest ideas for improvement. However, not everyone has a group of physiotherapy friends easily accessible for this purpose.

In my experience, the best people to ask for assistance with interviews are the following.

- *Business people* – preferably individuals with experience of conducting interviews. These professionals will give you valuable tips on greetings, body language, posture, rapport building and relaxing in interviews.

- *Peers* – it can be very useful to work with a group of fellow physiotherapy students/graduates, taking it in turns to question each other and benefit from each other's knowledge and expertise. It is likely you will all be preparing for interviews at the same time and have sourced different material regarding interviews. Also be sure to check out information on the student/graduate network of Interactive CSP. There is usually a great deal of discussion regarding what to expect at interviews and other graduates' previous experiences of a variety of interview formats, including helpful tips on preparing for the different types of interviews.

- *Tutors* – these individuals generally have broad clinical experience and are good at giving feedback. It is also more intimidating being interviewed by a tutor than a friend/peer. It is definitely worth asking your old or present tutors if they will go through a practice interview with you; they are usually more than willing. The only problem can sometimes be their availability or time, therefore as the saying goes – book early to avoid disappointment!

- *Physiotherapy clinicians* – you may be lucky enough to have a friend (yours or your family's) who is practicing physiotherapy. These people are in an ideal position to interview you. They have up-to-date knowledge of the skills, knowledge and attributes required by a practicing physiotherapist. The only difficulty is usually their availability. If you don't know anyone, don't worry, this is where your clinical placements may come in handy. Remember when you had to spend 4–6 weeks on placement being overfriendly to everyone? Wasn't it painful! It may have sucked at the time, but now you can take advantage of any telephone numbers you got at the end of the placement. You may feel a bit cheeky asking old clinical educators for help, but most professionals understand how worried you are before your first physiotherapy interview (after all, they've been there themselves!) and won't mind helping. Be assertive and polite and at the end of the day, remember, the worst they can say is no!

When practicing interview techniques, try to include a breadth of questions. The main topics to cover will be trust specific, job specific, personal attributes, clinical questions, experience and qualifications. Use "dummy" interviews to practice your communication skills, paying attention to both verbal and nonverbal methods of communication.

Interview tips

After you have entered the interview room, a firm handshake may help to break the ice and show you're a professional, and greeting the interviewer by name will help immediately to build rapport. Start by maintaining eye contact with the person to whom you are speaking and don't forget to balance eye contact amongst each of the interviewers. Practice articulating correctly, using succinct points and include those physiotherapy "buzzwords" you have brought into all your essays as a student (teamwork, evidence-based practice, problem solver, clinical reasoning). Most of us use filling words such as "erm" when we communicate, but these serve no purpose apart from disjointing a clear sentence. Try to increase consciousness of your use of filling words and limit their contribution in your sentences. Think about your posture and how you are sitting to make sure you look attentive and enthusiastic. Like most things, there is no "one size fits all" approach to making a good impression. It is important that you feel comfortable when entering the interview room so try to use whatever strategy works for you to put yourself at ease (picture your interviewer at home as a mum/dad, on the toilet or even in the nude if that works for you!). One of the main tips to a good performance is to relax.

Appearance

I'm sure you've been dressing yourself for years (well, I hope so, anyway!) and you are familiar with the kind of attire you are expected to wear for job interviews. However, I have heard from physiotherapy managers about applicants who turned up for interviews in jeans, unironed shirts and scruffy trainers so I think it is wise to include a briefing on appearance. When walking into an interview room, first impressions last, and the person conducting the interview will judge you initially on your appearance. This is an easy way to get the interview off to a good start so if you're a guy, either a suit or trousers, shirt (ironed!) and tie should do the trick. If you're a girl, smart trousers, long skirt, shirt, jumper or even a suit should impress. A smart appearance immediately conveys the message that you're sensible, responsible and professional, qualities needed to undertake the role of a physiotherapist. While wild hair, bitten nails and rugged stubble or overzealous make-up were commonplace in the students union, you're now about to enter the world of work so make an effort with your personal grooming. It's the little things that often count! The final point worth making is about *shoes*. It may be a mere coincidence but several interviewers with whom I have spoken *all* mentioned footwear. Do not be tempted to dig out your old scuffed work shoes or the trendy shoes your partner likes. It is time to opt for sensible, smart (you may say "boring"!) shoes, possibly even with a dab of that shoe polish you haven't seen since starting your degree. Just remember, as the old saying goes, "shoes maketh the man!" (or woman!).

On the day

So the day of the interview has finally arrived. Before now, you probably thought exam nerves were bad! In my own personal experience, I hadn't felt that level of anxiety since doing my driving test at 17! (sadly, for me, 10 years ago now). The point is that it is perfectly normal to be nervous and this can even help you achieve your best performance. Remember, all the other job applicants are feeling exactly the same as you and have the same fears of not performing to their potential. This may seem like common sense but try to relax and be yourself. Remember, as long as you've prepared properly, you can only do your best on the day. If that is not enough and you are not successful, then the job wasn't for you anyway. That advice may seem a bit lame if you really want the job, but having this attitude will save you putting too much pressure on yourself and decrease the risk of having one of the dreaded "mind blanks."

Ways of coping with stress

- Try some deep breathing exercises or meditation.
- Make a hot drink and watch your favorite TV show.
- Do some light exercise or sporting activity.
- Have a hot bath and listen to some relaxing music.
- Go round to a friend's house for a chat or watch a DVD.
- Consider your interview nerves in relation to the greater problems in society (e.g. civil war in Africa). This should make you feel like you have nothing at all to worry about.

Whichever way you cope with stress on the day, remember to smile, be polite, friendly, courteous, take time to think and give considered answers. In an interview situation it is perfectly acceptable to pause for a second to think or to ask the interviewer if you could return to answering a particular question later. Your case will not be hindered in any way by taking this action, but by blurting out the first thing that comes into your head, you might not do yourself any favors. A mistake of which I have been guilty is to keep talking until you have absolutely exhausted the subject (I'm sure I am not alone with this one). In my own mind I was ensuring that I "answered the question" by virtue of the fact that if you shoot enough bullets, one will probably hit the target. The problem with this approach is that you will either bore the interviewer with a great deal of erroneous information (and thus detract from time to answer other questions) or cloud your more pertinent points. In interviews, it is definitely quality over quantity when considering your answers. The other big lesson I've learned is when it comes to clinical questions, give the simple answers first. The major qualities interviewers try to assess are logical thinking and common sense. They are not expecting you to be a brain box in every specialty, but they do expect you to get the simple answers right and these are usually the ones that appear too obvious!

Conclusion

N. T. L Southorn

So there it is. I hope that this book has provided you with some helpful advice throughout your study. Once you become a fully fledged physiotherapist you will continue to learn and develop yourself – it is what makes this profession so interesting. The number of physiotherapists who do amazing things to show the more skeptical people of this world that physiotherapy is a leading profession in healthcare is ever increasing. Will you join the ranks of the truly inspirational clinicians?

Whatever you do as a practitioner, you should never forget the life you had with your friends at physio school; the good times and the bad all shape you and make you a better person.

To conclude – physio school is the start of something special in your life and the lives of every one of your patients … enjoy it!

Nick Southorn
(now a qualified physiotherapist)

A

Abduction, 46
AbilityNet members network (CSP), 18
Academic tutor, role of, 130
Access funds, 20
Accessory movement, 46
Accidents, 127
Accountability, 144
Active cycle of breathing techniques
(ACBT), components, 76
Active movement, 46
Activities of daily living (ADL), 50, 121
Acupuncture, 6, 54–55
Adduction, 46
Adrenoreceptor agonists, 96
Advances in Physiotherapy (journal), 67
Agenda for Change (NHS framework),
165
Aide mémoire, 59
see also Notes
American Drug Index, 98
American Physical Therapy Association
(APTA), 5, 7
Analgesic drugs, 95
Anatomy, 38–41
functional, 38, 54
mnemonics and chants, 39–40
study tips, 70–71, 71–72
visualizing, 38–39
Anecdotal evidence, electrotherapy, 65
Angiography, 116
Angiotensin-converting enzyme (ACE)
inhibitors, 96
Anterior cingulate cortex (ACC), 55
Antibiotic drugs, 96
Anticholinergic drugs, 96
Anticoagulant drugs, 96
Antidepressant drugs, 96
Antidiabetic drugs, 96
Antifungal drugs, 96
Antihypertensive drugs, 96
Anti-inflammatory drugs, 95
Antimicrobial drugs, 96
Antimuscarinic drugs, 96
Antiviral drugs, 96
Appeals, academic, 18–19

Appearance
job interview, 168–169
see also Uniform
Artefacts, assessment and, 51
Arterial blood gases (ABGs), 116
Articles, electrotherapy, 66–67
Assessment
cardiopulmonary, 74
integration into practice, 107–109
key points, 76
musculoskeletal, 47–50, 50–52, 53
neurologic, 86–87
pediatric, 114–117
techniques, 121, 165
Attentional processing, 104
Audit cycle, clinical, 136
Auscultation, 76
Australian Physiotherapy Association, 6
Autonomic nervous system, 85
Avoiders, pain and, 106

B

Back Pain Revolution (Waddell), 104
Balance, assessment, 87, 116
Banting, F., 137
Bed space, 78
Behavioral experiments, 108
Beliefs, 104–105
Berg Balance Scale, 116
Best, C.H., 137
Beta-blockers, 96
Biguanides, 96
Bindegewebsmassage (connective tissue
massage), 56
Biomedical approach, 102–103
Biopsychosocial approach, 101–110
clinical placement, 107–109
model of pain disability, 103–107
reasons for, 102–103
student wisdom, 109
Black and Minority Ethnic Members
Network (CSP), 18
Brain, 83–85
association areas, 73
Brainstem, 73
Breaks, 127

Breathing techniques, 56, 76
Brick wall approach, 53
British National Formulary (BNF), 98
Bronchi, 40
Bronchodilator drugs, 96, 97
Brushing, as treatment, 88
Bulk, muscle, 115
  assessment, 50
Bursaries, 20
Business people, job interviews and, 167

C

Calcium channel blockers, 96
Canadian Physiotherapy Association
    (CPA), 5
Cardiac arrest, 127
Cardiac rehabilitation, 138
Cardiopulmonary physiotherapy, 69–80
  clinical placement, 73–79
  theory, 70–73
Cardiopulmonary Physiotherapy (Jones &
    Moffatt), 72
Cardiorespiratory medicine, 97
Cardiovascular exercise, 89
Carpal bones, 39
Catastrophizing, pain and, 106
Caudad, 46
Cephalic movement, 47
Cerebral cortex, 83
Cerebral palsy (CP), 113, 118
Chants, mnemonics and, 39–40
Chartered Society of Physiotherapy (CSP),
    5, 7, 14–20
  benefits, 15–16
  fees, 15
  interactive (iCSP), 17–18
  membership, 14–15
  networks, 18
  portfolios and, 147–151
  publications, 67
  student representatives, 17
  students' officer, 16–17
Chest X-ray (CXR) analysis, 76
Childcare allowance, 20
Children *see* Pediatrics
Chiropodists, 90
Clinical audit cycle, 136
Clinical educator, role of, 130
Clinical Governance (NHS framework), 165
Clinical placement, 19, 119–132
  academic tutor, role of, 130

anatomy/physiology and, 43
biopsychosocial approach, 107–109
cardiopulmonary physiotherapy and,
    71, 73–79
clinical educator, role of, 130
costs, 20
elective, overseas, 19
FAQs, 129
hazards of, 77–79
information on arrival, 126–128
learning agreement, 128
marking criteria, 128–129
musculoskeletal physiotherapy (MSK)
    and, 58–59
neurologic physiotherapy and, 90–91
notes for, 43
pharmacology and, 98
preparation for, 120–121
  questions, 122
student wisdom, 79, 131–132
tips for, 75–77
Clinical reasoning, 70
Clinical semaphore, 52
Clothing
  job interview, 168–169
  see also Uniform
Cochrane database, 146
Cognitive behavioral therapies, 8
Collapse, 127
Communication, teams and, 145
Comparison study, 138
Compensation, exercise and, 58
Computed tomography (CT), 116
Computer access, 127
Conduct, student, 26–27, 30, 31
Confronters, pain and, 106
Connective tissue massage, 56
Consent, informed, 121
Continuous professional development
    (CPD)
  defined, 147–148
  see also Portfolio, CPD
Contraindications, 165
  electrotherapy, 65
Co-ordination, assessment, 87
Coping strategies, 106
  job interview stress, 168, 169
Coping Strategies Questionnaire (CSQ),
    140–141
CPD *see* Continuous professional
    development (CPD)

Cranial nerves
  functions, 84
  in order, 40
Critical care ward, 79
Cyclo-oxygenase (COX), 97
Cyriax treatments, 54
Cystic fibrosis (CF), 113, 116

D

Deep reflex nerve roots, 39
Degree-level study, 26
Dependants' allowances, 20
Dermatomes
  assessment, 87
  study tips, 85
Diabetes mellitus, 137
Dictionary of Physiotherapy (Porter), 46
Differential diagnosis, 86
Diseases, childhood, 113–114
Diuretic drugs, 96
Doctors, role of, 90
Domestic activities of daily living
  (DADLs), 50
Dose, of energy, 63
Double-blind approach, 138
Down's syndrome, 113
Drugs
  drug history (DH), 49
  see also Pharmacology
Duchenne muscular dystrophy, 113

E

Edema, assessment, 87
Educator, role of clinical, 130
Elective placements overseas, 19
Electrical stimulation, 89
Electrocardiograph (ECG), 116
Electroencephalography (EEG), 116
Electronic portfolios, 148
Electrophysical agents (EPA), 62
Electrotherapy, 61–68
  classification/terminology, 64
  defined, 62–64
  importance, 64
  model of, 63
  resources, 65–68
  student wisdom, 68
  study tips, 64–65
  top tips, 67–68
Electrotherapy: Evidence Based Practice
  (Watson), 66

Electrotherapy Explained (Robertson), 66
Emergency situations, 79
  equipment location, 127–128
  fire, 126
Emotional challenges, 112
Employment *see* Jobs
End feel, 115
Enteric nervous system, 85
Environment, exercise and, 57
Epidemiology, 85
Equipment, 10–11
  measuring, 11
  specialist, location, 122, 127–128
  tool box, 43, 89
Erector spinae muscles, 40
Ergonomics, 8
Etiology, 85
Evidence-based practice, 6, 145–146
Examinations, 31–33
  results, 158–159
Exercise therapy, 57–58
  physical activity, 108–109
  prescription, 46
  testing, 116
Expectancies, 105
Expectations
  lecturer, 27–29
  student, 30–31
Experimental research, 138–139
Expertise, 145
Extension, 47

F

Failure, 30, 32–33
'Fascial twist', 56
Fast passive stretch, as treatment, 88
Fear/avoidance model of pain,
  105–106
Fire emergencies, 126
Flags, system of, 52
Flexion, 47
Frameworks, NHS working practices, 165
Freshers' week, 11–12
Friendships, consolidating, 13
From Birth to Five Years (Sheridan), 113
Functional activity, 116
Functional anatomy, 38, 54
Functional magnetic resonance imaging
  (fMRI), 55
Funding, additional, 19–20
Fundraising, 18

G

Gait assessment, 51, 87, 116
Ganong's Review of Medical Physiology (Barrett), 10
Glasgow Biopsychosocial model for low back pain, 103
Goal setting, 106, 108, 117
Goniometers, 11, 46, 51, 122
Graduate opportunities, 159–160
Grants, NHS, 20
Graphesthesia, 116
Grays Anatomy (Standing), 9–10, 41
Group work, 13
Guidance for the Clinical use of Electrophysical Agents (CPS), 67
Gym ball, as treatment, 89

H

Handbooks, manufacturers', 67
Harland, N., 140–141
'Health coach', 8
Health Professions Council (HPC), 148
    re-registration, 152
Hippocrates, 6
Historical perspective, 5–7
    drug history (DH), 49
    past medical and surgical history (PMH), 49
    presenting condition (HPC), 48, 114
    social history (SH), 49–50
Hobbies, 50
Home circumstances, 50
Hospital, infection, 122
Houchen, L., 141–142
Human Histology (Stevens & Lowe), 41
Humeral fracture affects, 40
Hurt/harm, fear of, 105–106
Hydrotherapy, as treatment, 89
Hypervigilance, somatic sensations, 104

I

Ibuprofen, 97–98
Ice, as treatment, 88
Illness *behavior*, 104
Independent practitioner, 160
Industry, 160
Infection, hospital, 122
Information, 107–108
Informed consent, 121
Insulin, 96, 137

Insurance, 19
    professional and personal liability indemnity (PLI), 16
International classification of functioning, disability and health (WHO), 116
International organisations, 9
Internship, 160
Interviews
    semi-structured, 137
    strategy, 107
    structured, 137
    unstructured, 137
Interviews, job, 162–169
    appearance, 168–169
    format, 163
    practice with others, 167–168
    preparation for, 164–168
    questions
        clinical, 165, 169
        typical, 164
    stress, coping with, 168
    tips, 168

J

Jobs
    graduate opportunities, 159–160
    hunting for, 160–162
    social history and, 49
    see also Interviews, job
Joe Jeans Memorial Fund, 16
Joints
    compression, as treatment, 88
    function assessment, 115
Journal reviews, electrotherapy, 65

K

Knowledge, shared, 13
Knowledge and Skills (NHS framework), 165

L

Lancet (journal), 139
Language
    therapy, speech and (SLT), 91
    university, 25–26
Learning
    agreement, 128
    styles, 13
Legislation, 165
Lesbian, gay, bisexual and transgender (LGBT) members network (CSP), 18

Library access, 127
Literature, evaluating, 139
Littmann® Classic II, 75
Loop, 96
Low back pain, model for, 103

M

McKenzie treatments, 54
Magnetic resonance imaging (MRI), 116
    functional (fMRI), 55
Maitland treatments, 53
Maitland's Peripheral Manipulation
        (Hengeveld & Banks), 53
Maitland's Vertebral Manipulation
        (Maitland), 53
Manipulation, 47
Manual techniques, 6, 46, 90
Manual Therapy (journal), 67, 139
Marking criteria, clinical placement,
        128–129
Massage, 6, 58
Measuring equipment, 11
Medical Research Council muscle scale,
        115
Medical and surgical history (PMH),
        past, 49
Medscope, 75
Metoclopramide hydrochloride, 98
Misunderstandings, 108
Mnemonics and chants, 39–40
Mobilization, 47
    with movement (MWM), 56
Monoamine oxidase inhibitors, 96
Movement
    potential, 53
    range of (ROM), 51–52, 115
Mulligan treatments, 56
Multiple sclerosis (MS), 85–6
Muscle energy technique (MET), 55–58
Muscles
    assessment, 115
    bulk, 87, 115
    tone, 88, 115
Muscular dystrophy, 113, 118
Musculoskeletal physiotherapy (MSK),
        45–59
    assessment
        objective, 50–52
        subjective, 47–50
    clinical placement, 58–59
    clinical semaphore, 52

defined, 47
muscle energy technique (MET), 55–58
treatments, 52–55
Myofascial therapy, 56
Myotomes
    assessment, 87
    study tips, 85

N

Name badge, 124–125
Nerve conduction studies, 116
Nervousness
    clinical placement, 120, 131
    job interviews, 163, 169
Neurologic physiotherapy, 81–91
    assessment, 86–87
    basics, 83–85
    clinical placement, 90–91
    defined, 82
    management, 97
    presenting condition (PC), 82–83,
        85–86
    student wisdom, 90–91
    treatment, 88–89
    types, 83
*Neurological Physiotherapy: A Problem
        Solving Approach* (Edwards), 82
Neurology, 8
New Zealand Society of Physiotherapists
        (NZSP), 5, 7
Newsletters, electrotherapy, 67
Nonopioids, 95
Non-steroidal anti-inflammatory drugs
        (NSAIDs), 95, 97–98
Normal values, 77
Notes
    for clinical placement, 43, 74, 76, 126
    filing, 14
    for learning, 40
    noncontiguous, 13
    pharmacology, 98
    professional practice and, 145
Numerical Rating Scale (NRS), 49
Nurses, role of, 90

O

Objective assessment, 50–52, 121
    pediatrics, 115–117
Observation, 50–51
    research, 137–138
Occupational therapy (OT), 90

Opioids, 94, 95
Organizational knowledge, 165
Orthopedic medicine, 54
Osmotic drugs, 96
Outcome
    expectancies, 105
    studies, 138–139
Overdrafts, interest-free, 20
Overpressure, 47
Ovid database, 146

P

Pain
    assessment, 49
    disability, model of, 103–107
    exercise and, 57
    fear/avoidance model, 105–106
    management, 7, 97
Pain (journal), 139
Pain Management (Main), 104
Palpation, 41
Paper-based portfolio systems, 148, 149
Paradigm, 47
Parasympathetic nervous system, 85
Parkinson's disease (PD), 96
Passive movement, 47
Past medical and surgical history
        (PMH), 49
Pathology, 85
Patient-centred approach, 53
PebblePad, 148, 151
Pediatrics, 88, 111–118
    approach, to children, 112–113
    assessment, 114–117
    child development, 113
    diseases, childhood, 113–114
    treatments, 117–118
Peers, job interviews and, 167
Personal activities of daily living
        (PADLs), 50
Pharmacology, 93–99
    class system, 95–97
    clinical placement, 98
    drug knowledge, 97–98
Physical activity
    increase in, 108–109
    see also Exercise therapy
Physical Management in Neurological
        Rehabilitation (Stokes), 82, 114
Physical risk factors, 52
Physical Therapy Association, 7

Physical Therapy Reviews (journal), 67
Physical Therapy in Sport (journal), 67
Physiology, 41–43
    learning, 41–3
    movement, 47
    study tips, 72
    tool box, 43
Physiotherapists
    job interviews and, 167–8
    roles of, 7–8
Physiotherapist's Pocket Book (Kenyon &
        Kenyon), 10, 43, 98, 126
Physiotherapy
    defined, 5
    historical perspective, 5–7
Physiotherapy (online journal), 15
Physiotherapy Frontline (magazine), 15
Physiotherapy Research International
        (journal), 67
Physiotherapy for Respiratory and Cardiac
        Problems (Pryor & Prasad), 114
Physiotherapy Theory and Practice
        (journal), 67
Pilates, 56
Placebo effect, 63–64
Planned learning process model
        (CSP), 149–150
Play, therapeutic, 117
Podiatrists, 90
Portfolio, CPD, 147–154
    appearance, 148
    contents of, 149
    facts, 149–151
    material, ideas for, 153
    necessity of, 148
    online, 150, 151–152
    paper-based, 149, 152, 153
    steps, setting up, 152–153
Positioning, as treatment, 89
Positron emission tomography (PET), 116
Postgraduate study, 158–159, 160
Postisometric relaxation, 55
Posture, 51
Potassium sparing, 96
Potency, 95
Pre-registration courses, 158
Presenting condition (PC), 48
    history of (HPC), 48
    neurologic, 82–83, 85–86
Prevention, 8
Problem solving, 160

· Problem-based approach
assessment, 114–115
cardiopulmonary physiotherapy
and, 70
Professional and personal liability
indemnity insurance (PLI), 16
Professional practice, 144–145
Project development, 140
Proprioception, 116
assessment, 87
Proprioceptive neuromuscular facilitation
(PNF), as treatment, 89
Prostaglandin, 97
Psychologic risk factors, 52
Psychologists, 90–91
Psychosocial factors, assessment
mnemonic, 107
Publications (CSP), 67

Q

Qualitative research, 137–138
Quality of movement, 115
Quantitative research, 137
Questionnaires, 107

R

Randomized controlled trial (RCT),
138, 146
Range of movement (ROM), 51–52,
115
Ranson, C., 141
Reassurance, 107–108
Receptor agonist, 94
Receptor antagonist, 94
'Recipe' approach to treatment, 70
Reciprocal inhibition, 55
Recruitment agencies, 162
Red flags, 52
Reflection, 154–155
Reflexes, 115
Rehabilitation, 7, 8, 108, 138
Representation, 14–20
student, 17
Research, 136–142, 160
getting started, 139–140
papers as resource, 146
present day researchers, 140–142
project development, 140
types of, 137–139
Research ethics committee
(REC), 140

Resources, 13
Respiratory treatments, 117
Responsibility, 144
'Role play', 121
Rotator cuff muscles, 40
Rules of professional conduct, 144
*Rules of professional conduct and the
core standards for physiotherapy
practice* (CSP), 15, 26

S

Safety, exercise and, 57
Scheduling issues, 13
exercise and, 57
Scholarships, 19
Self-efficacy, 105, 107
Self-management, 105
Semaphore, clinical, 52
Semi-structured interviews, 137
Serotonin selective reuptake inhibitors
(SSRIs), 96
SIN factor (severity, irritability and
nature), 48
Single parent addition, 20
Skin assessment, 50
Slow passive stretch, as treatment, 89
SMART goals, 108, 128
Social history (SH), 49–50
Social life, 121
student wisdom, 14, 33
Social positioning, 24–25
Society of Orthopedic Medicine
(SOM), 54
Society of Trained Masseuses, 6
Somatic sensations, 104
Speech and language therapy
(SLT), 91
Spina bifida, 113
Spinal treatment, 54
Spirometry, 76, 116
Splinting, as treatment, 89
Sports medicine, 141
Steroids, 95
Stethoscope, 10–11, 74–75, 122
Strength, 115
training, 89
Stress, coping with, 106, 168, 169
Structured interviews, 137
Student Executive Committee
(SEC), 17
Student Representatives' Conference, 17

Study tips, 9, 35
    anatomy, 39–40, 71–72
    cardiopulmonary physiotherapy, 72–73
    dermatomes/myotomes, 85
    electrotherapy, 64–5
    individual, 13–14
    mnemonics and chants, 39–40
    physiology, 41–43, 72
    student wisdom, 33
Subjective assessment, 47–50
    pediatrics, 114–115
Success, seven steps to, 29–30
Sulphonylureas, 96
Surgical history (PMH), past medical
    and, 49
Sustained natural apophyseal glides
    (SNAG), 56
Sustained stretch, 55
Swelling, assessment, 87
Sympathetic nervous system, 85
Symptoms, 49

T
Tape measures, 11
Tapping, as treatment, 88
Targets, NHS, 165
Team work, 77, 145
    building skills, 13
    members, 127, 144
Telephone
    etiquette, 127
    numbers, 127
Test results, 77
Textbooks, 9–10, 66, 159
Therapeutic Exercise for Lumbopelvic
    Stabilization (Richardson), 58
Therapeutic Exercise: Foundations and
    Techniques (Kisner & Colby), 58
Therapeutic play, 117
Thiazide, 96
Thrombolytic drugs, 96–97
Tidy's Physiotherapy (Porter), 10

Tissue tension, 54
Tool box, 43, 89
Topics, breakdown of, 13
Traditional Chinese Medicine (TCM), 55
Travell, Janet, 56
Tricyclics, 96
Tutors
    job interviews and, 167
    role of academic, 130

U
Uniform, 11
    etiquette, 122–126
Unstructured interviews, 137

V
Vestibular stimulation, as treatment, 89
Veterinary physiotherapy, 8, 160
Vibration, as treatment, 88
Virchow, R., 102
Vocational rehabilitation, 7

W
Warm-up exercises, 57
Websites
    anatomy, 71
    electrotherapy, 62, 66
    Gray's anatomy for students, 10
    job hunting, 161–162
    medical equipment manufacturers, 73
    physiology, 72
    physiotherapy, 72–73
    Society of Orthopedic Medicine
        (SOM), 54
    'student consult' (Reed Elsevier), 40
Western medicine approach, 55
World Confederation of Physical Therapy
    (WCPT), 7

Y
Yellow flags, 52